BEATING STRESS,
ANXIETY
& DEPRESSION

Other titles by Jane Plant

Your Life in Your Hands: Understanding, Preventing and Overcoming Breast Cancer

The Plant Programme: Recipes for Fighting Breast and Prostate Cancer (with Gill Tidey)

Eating for Better Health: Recipes for Better Health (with Gill Tidey)

Understanding, Preventing and Overcoming Osteoporosis (with Gill Tidey)

Prostate Cancer: Understand, Prevent and Overcome

www.janeplant.com
www.stress-anxiety-depression-support.com

BEATING STRESS, ANXIETY & DEPRESSION

Groundbreaking Ways to Help You Feel Better

PROFESSOR JANE PLANT
and JANET STEPHENSON

piatkus

616.8522
Pla

PIATKUS

First published in Great Britain in 2008 by Piatkus Books
This paperback edition published in 2011 by Piatkus

A CIP catalogue record for this book
is available from the British Library.

ISBN 978-0-7499-3991-5

Text design by Paul Saunders
Illustrations by Rodney Paull
Typeset in ITC Stone Serif by
Action Publishing Technology Ltd, Gloucester
Printed and bound in Great Britain by
CPI Mackays, Chatham ME5 8TD

Papers used by Piatkus are natural, renewable and recyclable
products sourced from well-managed forests and certified
in accordance with the rules of the Forest Stewardship Council.

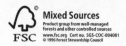

Mixed Sources
Product group from well-managed
forests and other controlled sources
www.fsc.org   Cert no. SGS-COC-004081
© 1996 Forest Stewardship Council

FSC

Piatkus
An imprint of
Little, Brown Book Group
100 Victoria Embankment
London EC4Y 0DY

An Hachette UK Company
www.hachette.co.uk

www.piatkus.co.uk

Contents

Jane would like to dedicate her contribution to the book to her parents Ralph and Marjorie Lunn, whose lives were so damaged by Ralph's depression. Janet dedicates her contribution to her children Jessie, Alex and Tasha.

Acknowledgements

We would like to thank Henry Haslam for his invaluable help in researching and writing the book. We are grateful to Judy Piatkus for agreeing to publish the book and to the editorial team at Little, Brown, led by Gill Bailey, for their support and advice. We particularly thank Jillian Stewart for her help in structuring the book. Professor Mustafa Djamgoz, neuroscientist and Professor of Cancer Biology at Imperial College, London is thanked for reading and commenting on Chapter 3 of the book. Thank you also to XiYu Phoon for preparing the first drafts of the diagrams.

Jane thanks her husband Peter and children Emma and Tom for all their help, support and encouragement, including commenting on draft chapters. Janet would like to thank Jessie for reading early drafts of the book. Thank you also to Xi Yu Phoon for preparing the first drafts of the diagrams.

Foreword

THE 20TH CENTURY SAW an unprecedented biological revolution that culminated in the dissection of the building blocks of 'life' itself, our genes. This is a spectacular application of science, particularly when we consider that it was only 50 years ago that the structure of DNA was first described by Watson and Crick. At about the same time, antimicrobials were first introduced for the treatment of life-threatening infections such as tuberculosis, and the birth of pharmacology as a subject enabled scientists and doctors to understand how drugs work in relation to our cells and organs and their function.

There can be no doubt that our much greater understanding of the structure and function of cells has created amazing opportunities to explain certain diseases – facilitating their early diagnosis and effective treatment. But it has also highlighted some important lessons that we need to learn.

First, our bodies are not driven by a series of simple biochemical pathways hence we cannot simply intervene at one end and expect a predictable outcome at the other. Secondly, our cells are not a simple 'bag' of chemicals that can be programmed. Instead we should consider them as a highly complex interacting set of molecules and 'scaffolding' that can be likened to the functioning of a city, with its people representing the molecules; its roads and buildings, the structures; and the power house of government, its nucleus, the control centre! Thirdly, apart from identical twins, every single human being on Earth is different. What is truly remarkable is that while humans have only 30,000 or so genes, the diversity of the human species can be explained by less than a 0.2 per cent variation in them. Thus understanding genes is only the start of unravelling the biological origins of health and disease. What is absolutely critical in most human diseases is how environment – both the external environment and the internal environment of our bodies – interacts with genes in ways that translate themselves into health or disease states.

At this point you may be wondering how all this is relevant to mood disorders such as anxiety and depression. The simple answer is that it highlights just how far we need to go before we understand how molecules and cells interact with each other to generate normal function and at what level(s) this becomes disturbed in diseases such as mood disorders. There can be no doubt that drug treatments for anxiety and depression can be of immense help – if, and it is a big if, the correct drugs are used based on accurate diagnosis – but, as this book highlights, the frequent failure to use good diagnostic procedures hinders their effective use and may in part explain the increasing level of side effects that patients are experiencing. The same problem may also limit the number of new drugs being discovered and developed. There is increasing evidence that drugs are only part of the answer for many patients suffering from stress, anxiety and depression.

So if drugs are not the sole answer to mood disorders, what is? In this fascinating book we are taken on a personal journey through the authors' own experiences of anxiety and depression and offered some interesting answers to that question. What is truly remarkable is their ability to gain such clear insight into their own difficulties and what they were able to do to resolve them and yet, at the same time, apply scientific rigour to try and understand and then convey what processes may be operating to create periods of depression and anxiety. In addition to a detailed description of their own and other patients' experiences with these disorders, Jane and Janet help the reader understand the complex nature of mood disorders and their various subtypes. Throughout the book they emphasise the importance of seeking medical help during the early stages, but also the importance of lifestyle and diet and how individuals can help themselves.

What comes over strongly is the general lack of understanding of how various aspects of brain function interact with the environmental and nutritional factors that are so closely related to the origins of these disorders. The authors do not 'duck' these issues but give clear guidance on environmental and nutritional interventions, underpinned by the latest scientific thinking about how they might work and why it is so important to think about the wider issues impacting on the brain – not just the management of symptoms through drug treatment.

This brings me back to the importance of understanding the complexity of how the brain works and the interdependence of one set of factors on another to determine both mood and psychiatric illness. It seems remarkable to me that the instruments that are still being used to measure whether a particular intervention, such as a drug, is effective or not are still in the relatively crude form of questionnaires, which are open to differing interpretation. The case for more quantitative methods of diagnosing and monitoring the effectiveness of treatment of anxiety and depression is well made in this book. Using new brain imaging techniques, it is now clear that the mere act of taking a tablet each day, even if it is a dummy drug or placebo, and believing that it works can have a beneficial influence on chemicals, metabolism and blood flow in the brain. It is remarkable that clinical trials of drugs to treat anxiety and depression often identify only small differences between the active agent and placebo – the active agent regularly accounting for less than 20 per cent of the response, and the remainder being attributed to 'non-specific' or 'placebo' responses. If almost 80 per cent of all patients' benefit from an intervention is as a result of the 'placebo' effect, then the placebo effect itself becomes an incredibly interesting phenomenon to explore scientifically.

If taking a dummy tablet every day can achieve this remarkable effect, then it is not difficult to imagine that environmental and nutritional factors can also have remarkable effects on the brain. A good example of this in anxiety and depression is the impact of the rural environment on human health and well-being; clinical trials demonstrating that such exposures may in some cases be superior to medication. Another example is the remarkable improvement in mood disorders brought about by a supportive family and a nurturing and positive attitude in doctors and other health-care workers.

Towards the end of the book the authors refer to the training of medical personnel and a need to listen to and understand patients' perspectives. There is relentless erosion of medical practitioners' time, frequently forcing them to rely on simple drug interventions, which adversely affects patient–health practitioner interactions. It is hardly surprising then that patients are voting with their feet by consulting complementary practitioners. From a patient's perspective this is entirely understandable if the complementary practitioner–patient interaction gives them the outcome that they seek in a more holistic way than can be achieved from orthodox medicine. So maybe what we should be trying to achieve is to draw together those aspects of creating and maintaining mental and physical 'health' (in contrast to emphasising curing disease). In essence this means more effort is needed to empower people suffering from mood disorders to help themselves with the appropriate interventions, and to enable them to alter their lifestyles accordingly and 'light up' those aspects of the brain that create a sense of health and well-being, mitigating against those of stress, anxiety and depression. Greater emphasis on these factors, with health practitioners engaging more widely with factors such as nutrition, environment, social and family structures would undoubtedly improve outcomes for the many millions of people who will suffer from a mood disorder at some point during their life, and can only benefit society as a whole.

This book is recommended to all sufferers of stress, anxiety and depression and their supporters, and health and social workers concerned with their treatment. It is also recommended to all those concerned with policy on the prevention and treatment of serious mood disorders.

Professor Stephen T. Holgate
MRC Clinical Professor of Immunopharmacology &
Honorary Consultant Physician, Southampton General Hospital;
Member of the Royal Commission on Environmental Pollution;
and board member of The Prince's Foundation for Integrated Health

Introduction

Vintery, mintery, cutery, corn,
Apple seed and apple thorn;
Wire, briar, limber lock,
Three geese in a flock.
One flew east,
And one flew west,
And one flew over the cuckoo's nest.

It MAY SEEM STRANGE to begin a book about beating stress, anxiety and depression with the nursery rhyme that inspired the title of one of the most dark and controversial books about mental illness, but *One Flew Over the Cuckoo's Nest* – and in particular the 1975 film version starring Jack Nicholson – has done a great deal to influence the public perception of mental illness. The film is set in a mental asylum and describes the lives of the disempowered patients who are forced to live in an uncaring and controlling regime. The mental asylum was in fact an allegory for the Soviet Union but the message that most people absorbed was that mental illness is a frightening experience that is outside our control and its onset heralds an inevitable downward spiral. One of the purposes of this book is to show just how wrong this widely held belief can be.

Our aim is to empower people suffering from stress, anxiety or depression – and their carers – to regain control of their treatment, their health and their lives. If you are reading this book it is likely that your life or the life of someone you love is already blighted by mental illness and you want to find help. The illness might be chronic low mood or stress, an intense anxiety state such as obsessive compulsive disorder (OCD), or unremitting black depression. Perhaps you have already talked to many doctors and other health professionals and read many books on the subject and are wondering why this one should make a difference. There are several reasons why we believe it will.

First, the book aims to take away the fear, helplessness and hopelessness we inevitably feel when suffering from mental ill health. It will help sufferers and their supporters to regain control of their lives by equipping them with the latest knowledge and evidence from mainstream medical and scientific literature, translated into accessible English. We believe that most people suffering the misery of a mood disorder, and their friends and family, want to understand what has gone wrong and what can be done to help. There is much new research that shows us how we really can make a difference to the prevention and treatment of mental illness. We believe that this should be available to everyone, not just scientists.

Secondly, we do not agree with the usual advice to 'keep taking your medication and eventually all will be well, because doctor knows best'. Indeed, we challenge many of the conventions in the treatment of mental illness, particularly the way that patients are prescribed medication without any diagnostic tests being carried out. You will therefore find lots of advice on getting the most out of your health professionals and health system, as well as an examination of the pros and cons of conventional, complementary and alternative treatments.

Training and expertise are also important. While you wouldn't necessarily expect your family doctor to have an in-depth understanding of the brain, you may be surprised to learn that we know of many psychiatrists, too, who have only a rudimentary knowledge of the brain and its workings. Indeed, it has been stated that psychiatrists are the only medical specialists who rarely look at the organ they treat.[1] We examine how training in this important speciality needs a better basis in science.

Third, this is not a 'single issue' book so it isn't solely about diet or learning new ways of thinking and it doesn't offer a simple one-size-fits-all answer for all mood disorders. We do not accept that the most popular form of antidepressant is the answer to all mood disorders or that cognitive behavioural therapy is the right treatment for everyone. We outline recent scientific findings which show that the human brain can be affected by many different problems and that a holistic approach – involving various types of medication (based on good diagnosis), nutritional therapy, exercise and emotional and social support – is likely to offer the best, most sustainable improvement in mood.

Like cancer and many other diseases, mental illness is a troubling subject but, unlike most physical illnesses, sufferers are often stigmatised. Few people understand what mental illness is, so it is viewed with fear and seen by many as shameful or embarrassing. But although mental illness is a subject that frightens most people this is not a frightening book – quite the opposite! We aim to replace the irrational fears and old wives' tales that influence our ideas about mental illness with a modern, rational understanding of what is really wrong with the workings of the brain when we suffer from mood disorders such as anxiety and depression.

Why, you might be wondering, are we equipped to write such a book?

This book was inspired by our own experiences as sufferers. We both know just how frightening mental illness can be: Jane experienced years of chronic anxiety after taking benzodiazepines to counteract the stress of cancer treatment, while Janet suffered from psychosis that began as post-natal depression and led to her spending several months in a frightening mental institution. We both remember clearly how helpless we felt at the time – part of a community that nobody wanted to know about. We are also all too well aware how little conventional medicine and psychiatry were able to help us. In the depths of our despair we could not believe that we would ever be well again. Thankfully, we are both now well and happy and want to share with you all we know about how we, and many others, have regained our health.

In addition to our personal experiences of mental illness we both have relevant professional experience and knowledge – Jane as a scientist and author of science-based health books and Janet as a practising psychologist.

Jane has worked for much of her career as a senior government and academic scientist and has received many awards for her contribution to science. She transformed thinking about the prevention and treatment of breast cancer with her best-selling book *Your Life in Your Hands*.[2] It describes how she overcame breast cancer, having suffered from the disease for a fifth time, using science-based dietary and lifestyle changes to complement her conventional treatment – changes that she believes saved her life. She has written best-selling books on osteoporosis[3] and on prostate and other types of cancer.[4] In 2005 she was elected as a Fellow of the Royal Society of Medicine for this work, and in the same year she qualified with a diploma in nutrition. She worked in a clinic in Wimpole Street, London, giving advice to patients on diet and lifestyle. She now works with Stress, Anxiety and Depression Support in Kew.

It was Janet's dreadful experience of psychosis, during which time she was never offered any counselling or therapy, which prompted her to become a psychologist. After many years of study and training she now works in an NHS hospital, running group sessions and holding one-to-one consultations. She also has her own successful private practice.

An important impetus for writing this book is our belief that for too long society has accepted mental illness without questioning why it occurs and what can be done to prevent the terrible toll that stress, anxiety and depression take on individuals and society as a whole. There is no doubt that we have all been persuaded to be too passive about our own mental well-being – to leave it to the professionals and, if we are ill, to 'keep taking the pills' and 'do what doctor says'.

Our advice is very different! It will empower you to take control of your mental health. Recent scientific advances have meant there is much to be optimistic about. Rapid advances in neuroscience, based on the latest non-invasive techniques of brain imaging, are contributing to a much improved understanding of the brain–mind–body system and what can go wrong to cause mental illness. Some of the very latest methods of imaging allow the distribution of chemicals in the brain to be mapped so precisely that it has been said that a single thought can be followed. This new information, combined with earlier experimental and observational research, not only identifies some of the key biological–biochemical mechanisms involved, but is also leading to an understanding of the interplay of social, environmental and biological factors that are involved in anxiety and depression. This book will show you how to use this information to help prevent and treat stress, anxiety and depression.

In Part One we begin by describing our own experiences of treatment in the UK National Health Service (NHS), which will help you understand how things can go wrong – and right – with various forms of treatment. We then look at the different types of anxiety and depression and review new models of the brain–mind–body system based on brain scanning and imaging techniques and other research. We also outline the latest thinking on how individuals become vulnerable to anxiety and depression and the factors that trigger these illnesses.

In Part Two we consider the treatments for mood disorders, many of which continue to be used on an empirical or 'suck it and see' basis. Mental illness is one of the few remaining serious illnesses still diagnosed simply on the basis of a clinical interview using subjective criteria. This is despite the fact that there are now more rigorous scientific approaches available to diagnose and treat sufferers. We look at these in detail.

Conventional drug treatments are a vital issue and we examine their use from a personal as well as professional perspective. Other chemical interventions, such as herbal treatments and targeted amino acid therapies, are beginning to be more widely used and their efficacy is discussed. We also examine the value of psychological talking therapies such as cognitive behavioural therapy (CBT) and psychodynamic counselling (PDC) in helping people to identify the root causes of their condition and to develop coping strategies. We then outline the fascinating methods that can be used to access the emotional mind – which is not reached by words and language – in order to heal our emotional and mental scars.

We go on to discuss controversial physical treatments such as electroconvulsive therapy and neurosurgery for mental disorder, which, thankfully, are beginning to be overtaken by far more gentle, science-based methods that use magnetism and pacemaker-like implants in the brain respectively.

How you live your day-to-day life is clearly of crucial importance and the lifestyle factors we suggest in Part Three are designed to help reduce stress levels, especially chronic stress, which can be a key factor in precipitating mental illness.

Everyone is aware that diet plays a vital part in our physical health but what is less well known is that we can also improve our mental health by improving our diet – and there is a great deal of new evidence to show this. Did you know, for example, that some scientists now believe that many people's mental illness may be associated with simple lithium deficiency because of the food and drinks they consume? Many leading doctors and scientists now consider that nutrition is vital to the brain and its proper functioning and that the right kind of food can dramatically improve outcomes for people with stress, anxiety and depression, including serious illnesses such as bipolar disorder. Our ten easy-to-follow food factors will help you incorporate the latest science-based advice on diet into your daily life to help prevent such illnesses.

We think you'll find the case histories useful, as they provide an insight into how various factors affect sufferers and how these people have managed to recover their health.

In the last chapter of the book we argue for a new paradigm to reduce the toll that mental illness increasingly takes on individuals and society as a whole, and, finally, to take the emphasis back to you, we provide 12 key golden guidelines for beating stress, anxiety and depression.

It is our hope that this book will serve two purposes. First, we want it to be directly useful to you, the reader. If you happen to be that one in five or six people whose life has been affected by anxiety or depression we hope that the information in this book will help you to overcome your illness and lead a more fulfilling life.

Secondly, it is vital that the book ignites a debate. Compelling evidence from the peer-reviewed scientific and medical literature has led us to the inescapable conclusion that mental health systems – and in particular that of the UK, which has staggered on almost unchanged for half a century – need a dramatic overhaul to bring treatment up to the standards of the best cancer centres in the NHS or to the very best private mental health clinics in the USA. Moreover, providing patients with advice on lifestyle and dietary changes, as is common in the case of heart disease or diabetes, could greatly improve outcomes. It is also imperative that governments and society as a whole do far more to reduce the numerous sources of stress that impinge on our lives – sources as diverse as exposure to neurotoxic substances, badly designed housing and towns, and a lack of access to green space for exercise and leisure. Much suffering could be prevented if the evidence brought together in this book is heard and acted upon with urgency.

Above all we hope that the information that the book contains will help you if your life, or the life of someone you love, is badly affected by stress, anxiety or depression. Remember that the brain is a truly amazing organ which, unlike most organs of the body, has an incredible ability to be shaped and reshaped – and therefore it can be healed.

Jane and Janet

HOW TO USE THE BOOK

The book is in three parts. If you are presently suffering from stress, anxiety or depression, we suggest you begin by reading Chapter 1, which features our stories. These demonstrate that we have 'been there' ourselves and that although we are fully recovered we understand how you might be feeling now. We hope they will also give you encouragement. You should then find the next chapter (Introducing Stress, Anxiety and Depression) helpful as it describes the main types of mood disorders. Chapter 3 examines the new understanding we have of the brain–mind–body system and what goes wrong with it to cause mental illness. In particular it will help you to understand how drug treatments work. It is a complex subject, however, so you may want to read this chapter and Chapter 4, which examines some of the main risk factors for mood disorders, when you are feeling a little better.

Part Two of the book, which examines all the various types of treatment and their effectiveness, will help you assess those which may be appropriate to you. When you are on the road to recovery, we suggest you proceed to Part Three to find out what you can do in terms of lifestyle and diet to help treat your illness and prevent it coming back.

Finally, Chapter 11 should be of interest to all those affected by mental illness, as well as those working in this field. It sets out our recommendations for what we need to do as a society to help prevent mental illness and in particular how health systems need to be improved. If it encourages you – even at the smallest most personal level – to highlight the case for better health care for sufferers then we will have gone some way to helping those suffering from mental illness.

Part One

UNDERSTANDING
STRESS, ANXIETY AND
DEPRESSION

In this section of the book we help you to understand what mood disorders are, what causes them and why some people seem to be more vulnerable than others. We explain, in simple terms, how the brain works and what can go wrong to cause you to suffer from stress, anxiety or depression.

Chapter One

In Two Minds

W<small>E BEGIN BY TELLING</small> you our own stories so you will understand why we care so passionately about helping people whose lives are badly affected by anxiety, depression, stress or even just persistently low mood. You may feel, as we did, that you will never regain your health but, as our stories illustrate, although you might be seriously ill now, it is possible to make a full recovery.

JANE'S STORY: A CASE OF ANXIETY

Storm clouds brew

On a warm, sunny afternoon in 1993 I set out for the hospital where I had been treated for breast cancer. Two weeks before, I had undergone a minor operation to remove a cancerous lymph gland in my neck. This was the third time my cancer had recurred following a mastectomy to remove my left breast in 1987, and I was now returning to hospital because a large lump had appeared in the scar where the cancerous node in my neck had been removed.

When the oncologist examined my neck and told me my cancer was back yet again my heart sank and I could see nothing but a painful and miserable end ahead. I agreed to begin chemotherapy as soon as possible, but I could not think how I was going to get through the next few days, with my mind racing with its grim imaginings. I was prescribed a tranquilliser but this did nothing to calm me, so I asked for something stronger. That is when I was prescribed a strong benzodiazepine drug called lorazepam (Ativan). What I didn't realise was that the drug I had been prescribed was highly addictive and had been used in the past on Russian dissidents to help them sleep; when these 'sleeping tablets' were withdrawn, it could be guaranteed that many would commit suicide. Little did I know then that it would cause me many years of anguish.

Pills, pills and more pills

During the next six months I hardly thought about the little blue pills I was taking – I was simply pleased that they would knock me out after chemotherapy – but then I started to have problems. About two months after the end of chemotherapy, my cancer had disappeared and I was back at work. Then, while talking to two colleagues, I noticed that they appeared to have luminous electronic worms emerging from their heads. When these strange symptoms began to occur more frequently, I decided that the pills were the cause and I would stop taking them. My solution was simply to leave them behind on my next weekend trip to London with my husband Peter. The first night without them was totally sleepless and the second was worse – my intellect seemed fine but I was frightened and anxious. Eventually Peter decided I needed medical help and took me to a walk-in medical centre nearby. The doctor initially thought I was suffering from stress as a result of my cancer and its treatment, but when I mentioned lorazepam she explained how addictive the tablets are and that my symptoms were withdrawal symptoms. She advised gradual and supervised withdrawal.

Despite the doctor's advice I decided to use my will power and simply stop taking the tablets. After all, I'd successfully overcome breast cancer and I'd never been addicted to anything before – I'd never smoked cigarettes or tried cannabis and rarely drank alcohol. I persisted in not having any more tablets but I became worse, especially during the early morning. One of the worst things was the incessant thought, a particularly cruel symptom of the mental state I was in, that everyone, including my husband and children, would be better off without me. Eventually I had to be taken to hospital where Peter was told I would have to have one-to-one nursing for six months.

In hospital, I was treated with a high dose of tricyclic antidepressants. The side effects were appalling: my eyes felt as if they would burst, my hands shook uncontrollably and my mouth was permanently dry in a way that was not eased by drinking any amount of water. I was also still suffering from the effects of the benzodiazepine withdrawal, with endless panic attacks when my heart would race and I would suffer palpitations and sweats. I found the hospital environment frightening and after a week I managed to convince my doctors that I could be allowed home safely. I stopped taking the antidepressants as soon as I was allowed out but I remembered that I had the remains of a prescription for what I thought was a weaker type of benzodiazepine, nitrazepam (Mogadon), which I had been prescribed while being treated with radiotherapy. I took two that night and slept well. I decided this was my way out and I'd found a way of coping. My doctor agreed to prescribe these for me and I was able to cope for a few years.

The last straw

In 1999 we began to suffer the loss of several friends and family, culminating in my mother's death in 2001. I was an only child and I now felt orphaned and bereft, despite being middle-aged with three grown-up children.

The last straw was when Peter was suddenly taken ill with tachycardia, a heart condition that is not normally life-threatening but appears very frightening. I had confronted my own mortality but never Peter's. When I returned alone from the hospital to a dark empty house I felt desolate. Despite taking my two nitrazepam tablets, I couldn't sleep. After pacing around, thinking of phoning friends and then concluding it was far too late, I decided to have some of Peter's malt whisky. When I came round the next morning, I found

I'd emptied the bottle. The same thing happened the following two nights while Peter was in hospital. When he was discharged three days later with a relatively clean bill of health I should have stopped taking the alcohol, but it eased the fear that Peter was going to die and leave me alone.

Over the next year, I would worry endlessly during the night and used alcohol to get some sleep. I woke up feeling depressed and totally worthless. I would go to work, although I was aware I was becoming less and less effective. The same thoughts would go round and round in my head and I would go over the same ground again and again, obsessed with my own problems and clinging to anyone who would listen to me. At the weekend I would try to treat my anxiety with remedies ranging from St John's wort teas to rhodiola root to kava kava but these herbal remedies were unable to counteract the state I was in as a result of my benzodiazepine and alcohol abuse.

When I was suffering from cancer, I had found that most people were incredibly supportive and helpful. The response to this illness was very different – when I appeared anxious and down, many people simply took advantage of the situation. I can understand why – I'd worked with people with an alcohol or drug problem in the past and I'd shown them no understanding or sympathy. I simply thought they should pull themselves together. It was impossible for me to imagine how badly people who abused alcohol, especially when combined with drugs such as benzodiazepines, could feel.

Eventually I discussed my problems with my doctor. Unfortunately he decided I was depressed and prescribed more of the antidepressant dothiepin without indicating the importance of giving up alcohol. I simply added the dose to my alcohol and nitrazepam, making matters worse. When I told my doctor that the dothiepin wasn't working he switched me to various selective serotonin reuptake inhibitors (currently the most commonly prescribed form of antidepressants) but these all caused hallucinations. He then referred me to a psychiatrist, who duly prescribed more pills that proved just as useless as the others and when I asked about counselling, told me to look on the Internet! He was, he said, unable to recommend anyone personally.

The way out

One afternoon, I was so ill that Peter called an ambulance. I was seen by a wonderful doctor who took a detailed case history. He was very reassuring and wisely helped me to find counselling and therapy, which put me on the road to recovery. The counselling was a great support and it helped me to see that the appalling withdrawal symptoms I was still suffering were due to the benzodiazepine withdrawal rather than some emotional problem. It made me realise that the only person who could help me was me.

I decided to research the problem for myself. I had almost certainly saved myself from dying of cancer using my scientific knowledge and experience so I could see no reason why I shouldn't be able to fight this too. Starting from the premise that I was suffering from withdrawal from benzodiazepine, I began looking for information on the Internet. In no time at all I confirmed that all my symptoms fitted this diagnosis and that the problems were due to the effects of benzodiazepines on something called the GABA receptor in the brain (which helps increase tranquillity). None of the antidepressants I'd been given had helped because all of them worked on different neurotransmitter systems.

I quickly learned that alcohol worked at the GABA receptor, explaining why I had problems with alcohol and why others, once treated with benzodiazepines, are at risk of becoming alcoholics. Obviously I wanted to find something more benign than either benzodiazepines or alcohol. I then discovered that an amino acid called taurine worked at the GABA receptor. I also learned which foods it was in and that it could be purchased from health food shops. At last, I thought I had found something that might help me. After a little more research I decided that in addition to taurine pills I'd take 5-HTP, the precursor of serotonin (see page 125).

After just a day I began to feel better and by the end of the week I was much more able to cope. The supplements did not make me feel drugged or sedated – just much more normal. While I doubt I will ever be the person I was before my cancer and treatment with benzodiazepine – I still react more to stress than before – I generally cope well. I take taurine now only if I feel stressed or if I sense the beginnings of an anxiety state. I have recommended taurine to several people with alcohol problems, who use it to good effect to help deal with their cravings – though they need other support as well.

After feeling better for a few weeks, I discussed my findings with a friend and colleague who is an eminent neurobiologist. His response was, 'What a good idea. I wonder why nobody has thought of that before.' But I was to discover that it had been thought of before (we examine amino acid therapies on page 125).

Looking back, I realise how fortunate I was compared to others in a similar state. My family and most of my friends remained supportive over the years and, probably because of that support, I managed to come out the other side of my illness and without becoming an alcoholic, which unfortunately happens to many sufferers.

JANET'S STORY: A CASE OF SEVERE POST-NATAL DEPRESSION AND PSYCHOSIS

What happened to Janet 25 years ago is particularly distressing. We would like to reassure you, however, that the vast majority of cases of post-natal depression do not lead to psychosis and are readily treated using modern therapies.

The nightmare begins

My first child, Jessie, was born in 1982. I had been married for about a year and lived with my husband, Jonathan, in a small flat. I'd attended classes held by the National Childbirth Trust, read numerous books about babies and childbirth and had decided that I would like to have a natural birth, in hospital but with no medical intervention. Unfortunately, labour went on for 18 gruelling hours but when, eventually, Jessie was born I fell in love with her instantly and felt a sense of elation that lasted for the next few weeks.

On my return home, my relationship with Jessie continued to flourish, but she slept for only a couple of hours at a time and I was becoming exhausted. Then the Falklands War began and my father, who was in the Royal Navy, was posted to London and came to stay with us in our tiny flat. Discussions about the war added to the stress and with hindsight I realise that I was beginning to suffer from depression.

When it transpired that the war was going to be protracted, my mother also moved in with us and I began to feel more and more stressed. I should have discussed my feelings, but Jonathan had started a new job and I was reluctant to burden him with my troubles.

The overcrowding problem was solved when my parents bought our flat, allowing us to move to somewhere with more space. However, by this time I felt very resentful and isolated and was exhausted by spending all night every night trying to persuade Jessie to go to sleep. I was also eating as little as possible in order to lose weight. Looking back, it's clear I was undernourished, especially as I was breast-feeding, and was probably deficient in a lot of essential nutrients.

Tipped into psychosis

Despite moving into our new home I was beginning to feel more and more lost, and when, at our house-warming party, a friendly neighbour, who seemed genuinely pleased that we'd moved in, offered me a puff of a joint he'd rolled I felt grateful and accepted. This was a big mistake. I'd never been a dope smoker, although I had tried it on two or three previous occasions. I was avoiding alcohol because I knew it would affect my breast milk but I didn't realise that cannabis would do the same. I was so depressed and debilitated that even a small amount had a strong effect on me. Rather than relaxing me, as I'd hoped, it made me feel strange, tearful and paranoid. That night seemed to go on for ever – I was scared, lonely and full of a sense of doom. Finally, in a panic, I started phoning friends and family, asking them to stay on the line as long as possible because I was so afraid. When a few of them came round to make sure I was OK it was obvious they thought I'd gone mad.

The following few hours were a bit of a blur. When I looked at people's faces I saw what to me seemed like evil. Then an amazing light seemed to swamp me, a luminous light I'd never experienced before. It lit up every blade of grass and I thought it was sent from heaven to help me. It was nothing like sunlight or electric light and it seemed to 'connect' everything in nature, including myself. The memory of this kept me going for the next few months. Of course, although neither I nor my doctors realised it at the time, all these symptoms, from paranoia to hallucinations, are typical of cannabis psychosis. People might find it difficult to believe that all this happened as a result of smoking a single joint of cannabis, but remember how exhausted, debilitated and depressed I was at the time.

A strange awakening

The next thing I knew I was put into a police van and taken to a grim-looking building. When I awoke I was in an unfamiliar room and had no idea what time of day it was or where I was. That first day in the hospital was petrifying. When I ventured out of my room, feeling like a zombie from all the medication I had been given, I found my way to where lunch was being served. As I went into the dining room, pills were being given out. I simply copied everyone else and held out my hand, only to be given various tablets and watched while I swallowed them with some water. Jonathan came to visit that day and said Jessie was fine but I couldn't see her for a while. Not surprisingly, I became very upset and I was then bundled into a little room and injected with what I later found out were the antipsychotic drugs Stelazine and Largactil, which are normally used to treat schizophrenia.

Escape and punishment

A few days later I determined to make my escape. I stole a fellow patient's bicycle and headed for the exit of the secure hospital. After a while, I abandoned the bicycle and got on a bus. I hoped nobody would ask me for money. They didn't. When I eventually reached my father-in-law's home, the look on his face when he saw me was enough to make my heart sink. I didn't get to see Jessie, who I was told was asleep, and after a short time Jonathan and his brother drove me back to the hospital.

My medication was now increased and I was moved to a locked ward that contained about 16 beds. I was among the long-term mentally ill and for the first time encountered catatonic schizophrenics.

The mood among the patients changed from stupor to aggression within short periods of time, and the staff remained behind mirrored glass through which they could see us but we couldn't see them. I was as terrified of the staff as I was of the patients.

Every evening Jonathan came to see me in the visitors' room, always talking first to the nurses before he talked to me. I realised that I was among a population that had no rights – we were humiliated, humbled and degraded. I felt paralysed and feared that I would become like the rest of them. All the time my medication was being increased and I knew that if nothing changed I would go mad – and I began to wonder whether I had already. I was in a constant state of terror, which was compounded at night by the cries of other patients ricocheting around the walls of the hospital courtyard. I resolved to leave the place but my attempt was in vain and ended in my being hurled into a padded cell.

The next day, Jonathan appeared as normal. I begged him to get me out of the hospital and shortly afterwards I was moved. The new hospital allowed more freedom, but a similar system based on fear prevailed and I began to feel hopeless. It was then suggested that I could have electroconvulsive therapy (ECT) which, we were informed, can have remarkable effects. I told Jonathan that I would never forgive him if he signed the papers giving permission.

I was kept on strong medication, but Jonathan realised that I was becoming more and more dejected. In desperation, he decided to contact the National Childbirth Trust, where we had attended ante-natal classes. He was told that another woman had recently suffered from the same symptoms and had been successfully treated with hormones. He was advised to read *Depression after Childbirth* by Dr Katharina Dalton,[1] which documents the case histories of several women who had suffered from post-natal depression. One of the case histories, about a woman who had had post-natal psychosis, was remarkably similar to my story.

Jonathan contacted Dr Dalton who told him that my post-natal decline was not uncommon and that I should take natural progesterone. When he told the psychiatrist at the hospital that having sought alternative medical advice he now believed my problem to be hormonally based it was suggested that he was becoming unstable too. Nevertheless he managed to get me discharged for a weekend and took me to see Dr Dalton. She did a blood test which showed that I was indeed severely deficient in progesterone.

The treatment was effective and I gradually recovered my health. I was advised that I would be at great risk of recurrent mental health problems if I had more children. Dr Dalton assured me, however, that if I were treated with progesterone immediately following the birth of any more babies I would be fine. Happily, I went on to have two more children and, having had progesterone injections following their births, had no further problems.

A few words of reassurance

This chapter has highlighted problems caused by the over-prescription of addictive drugs, the use of recreational drugs and repeated misdiagnosis. We would like to reassure you that all these problems can be avoided. Most doctors are now more aware of the dangers of over-prescribing drugs such as benzodiazepines and they are less likely to be given for more than a few weeks. In Chapters 5 to 8 we describe what needs to be done to improve the treatment of the mentally ill, including introducing some better approaches to diagnosis and treatment, which are already available in the best private clinics.

Chapter Two

Introducing Stress, Anxiety and Depression

LET US SAY AT THE outset that it is only human to be anxious or unhappy sometimes, for example if we have an important examination to sit or have recently undergone a divorce. It is normal to experience strong emotions at such times and in most people the feelings resolve once the stressful event has passed or, in the case of separation or loss, given time and support. Such natural emotions should not be regarded as mental illness and do not normally require medication. Indeed some eminent psychiatrists believe that sadness that is a normal reaction to losses and other adverse life events is being medicated into oblivion as 'depression'.[1]

However, many people in the modern world are affected by some form of mood disorder – for some it may be a persistent low mood that simply will not lift, for others it is a more serious anxiety state or depression that can be debilitating. Many people also visit their doctor because they are suffering from stress. Stress is very pervasive in modern life, and although it is a natural part of all our lives, it can lead to mental and physical illness if it persists and we don't learn to adapt and cope.

Anyone who has suffered from mental illness knows that it is much more than concern or unhappiness about some element of their life, and that it is not simply a character flaw or weakness that you can just snap out of. If you are a sufferer you will find it reassuring to know that, in fact, most conditions reflect an underlying physiological disorder – just as much as heart disease or diabetes – and that once diagnosed correctly most conditions can now be treated effectively.

If you suffer from anxiety or depression and perhaps are unable to hold down a job because of it, you are certainly not alone. Throughout the West such illnesses now affect more and more people and are a far greater cause of disability than cancer. In Britain, for example, 40 per cent of all disability (as indicated by the number of people in receipt of Disability Benefit) is due to mental illness (the vast majority of which is stress, anxiety or depression) compared to 2 per cent for cancer.[2] Mental illness does not discriminate – it strikes young and old, rich and poor, and men and women of all races – but few people willingly admit to having suffered from it. Part of the reason for this is that there is a general lack of awareness among the general public that mood disorders are very different conditions to psychotic illnesses such as schizophrenia.

Muddying the waters

Much of the fear and stigma surrounding mental illness is the result of sensationalist media reporting of violent incidents involving people suffering from schizophrenia. These events are rare, and schizophrenia accounts for only a small proportion of mental illness, yet the column inches devoted to the topic adversely affect society's attitude towards the far more common forms of mental illness such as anxiety and depression.

Schizophrenia is usually described, incorrectly, as a form of split personality, as if the condition reflects some sort of Jekyll and Hyde state. Schizophrenia is a serious psychotic disorder but the 'split' is, in fact, between the mind and reality. Untreated, victims can suffer from false fears of persecution or paranoia and disturbed sensory sensations, including hearing voices. Effective drug treatments for schizophrenia began to be developed in the 1950s and it is now treated so effectively that most sufferers can live reasonably normal lives in the community. Schizophrenia appears in cultures around the world and strikes roughly one half to one per cent of most populations.[3] Contrary to the impression given in the media, it is not on the increase (although there is some evidence that the rate of psychosis increases in cannabis users).

A growing problem

In contrast to the small percentage of people who suffer from schizophrenia, the number of people affected by mood disorders such as anxiety and depression is overwhelming and the incidence continues to increase. As many as one in six UK citizens and one in five Americans will be affected at some time in their lives.[4] It has been said that in Britain today chronic anxiety and crippling depression are the biggest causes of human misery, but the problem is hidden because of the shame and stigma still associated with these illnesses.[5] This is despite the fact that people suffering from anxiety and depression are highly unlikely to harm anyone except themselves.

THE SIGNIFICANCE OF STRESS

Stress alone can cause us health problems and, if we fail to adapt or cope, intense or chronic stress can lead to anxiety or depression.[6] The word 'stress' is short for distress and is derived from a Latin word meaning to pull apart – and most people who have been subjected to stress will be able to relate to this description. In 2005–2006 alone almost half a million people in Britain in employment believed they were experiencing work-related stress that was making them ill, and one in six of all workers thought their job was extremely stressful,[7] but stress is related to many other factors besides work.

Doctors define stress as the disruption of 'homeostasis', which is our internal metabolic equilibrium or balance. Our inner equilibrium must be maintained in relation to the ever-changing physical and social environment in which we live because it is essential to our survival, and consequently various feedback loops have evolved to maintain our physiological processes within the narrow range that is compatible with life. Some of the ways we adapt and cope with physical stress are easy to understand and are well known. For example, if it becomes too hot we perspire to evaporate water to keep us cool, and if we become dehydrated the brain stimulates us to take in fluid by making us feel thirsty so our equilibrium is maintained. However, the effects of stress from ongoing pain or pressure, whether physical or emotional, are less widely understood – though the impacts on our body (such as high blood pressure) and mind (such as anxiety and depression) can be substantial if we do not learn to adapt and cope.

In the next chapter we look at the effects of stress on the body and mind from a scientific point of view, based on the evidence of animal experiments (see pages 63–5). Here we consider some of the practical aspects of stress to help us to understand its effects on our mental health.

Stress and mental health

Many of us think of stress as purely negative. In fact we all need some degree of stress, interest and excitement in our lives if we are to function well, but problems arise when stress levels exceed our individual ability to cope. A human function curve (see page 24) – originally developed to explain the difference between good stress (eustress, defined by Richard Lazarus in 1974 as stress that is healthy or that gives one a feeling of fulfilment) and bad stress (distress) – can be used to understand the role of stress in anxiety and depression.[8]

The up slope and the down slope

On the up slope of the curve, performance improves in proportion to arousal, and mind and body activity is restored by sleep and relaxation. In this state, the equilibrium of the brain–body–mind system is maintained. Once an individual's ability to cope is exceeded, however, effort on the down slope continues but performance deteriorates and levels of circulating stress hormones start to increase. This results in dysphoria – feelings of emotional and mental discomfort and restlessness. This condition, if it becomes chronic, can contribute to the development of eating disorders and/or drug and alcohol abuse, and

The human function curve

Based on Nixon, P. *The Practitioner* 1979 and Posen, D. B. 'Stress management for patient and physician', *The Canadian Journal of Continuing Education*, April 1995

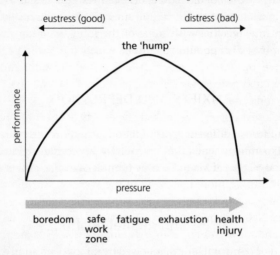

is generally differentiated from depression by a feeling of agitation. In this situation sleep, which normally is restorative, deteriorates and other indications of mind–body problems increase.

People may not recognise their negative emotional state or respond appropriately, ignoring or suppressing it (an increasingly common condition known by doctors as alexithymia), until exhaustion and finally breakdown or uncoping stress is established (see Chapter 3).[9] On the down slope, cognitive ability (conscious intellectual activity such as thinking, reasoning or learning) is impaired and in an exhausted state negative emotions including despair and hopelessness take over, often with no basis in reality.

There is strong evidence of a considerable interplay between stress hormones, including cortisol, and cognitive function, whereby cortisol affects cognitive function but cognitive processing also affects cortisol secretion.[10] This is the psycho-biochemical basis of cognitive behavioural therapy, which is just one of the powerful therapies now available to help sufferers (see Chapter 7).

Everyone will have a different curve and in vulnerable individuals the beginning of the down slope will begin at lower levels of stress.

Moreover, for some people it will be one episode of intense stress (for example, the loss of a loved one) that tips them over onto the down slope. There are major differences between one person and another in the kinds of situation that they find stressful. This is discussed further in Chapter 4, together with some of the most important causes of stress that can disrupt our equilibrium.

ANXIETY AND DEPRESSION

There are several different types of mood disorder. Standardised criteria for diagnosing mental illness generally, known as the DSM (Diagnostic and Statistical Manual), have been developed by the American Psychiatric Association, but many of the symptoms of the different types of anxiety and depression are overlapping. One of the big divisions that is usually made is between anxiety states and depression. In the UK and most Western countries, anxiety disorders are the commonest type of mental illness, followed by mixed depression and anxiety, and then depression alone.[11] These conditions can last a lifetime, though usually with long periods of remission.

Anxiety states

Many people with an anxiety disorder will suffer from more than one condition,[11] and anxiety is frequently associated with depression and substance abuse. Some of the most important psychological, emotional and physical symptoms are outlined below. Most anxiety disorders will include some of these symptoms, in different combinations and intensities.

Common symptoms of chronic anxiety

There are three main groups of symptoms: psychological symptoms such as obsession and worry; interpersonal problems, especially the need for reassurance; and physiological symptoms such as palpitations (racing heart). These can manifest in the following ways:

- Being fearful and apprehensive
- Feeling restless
- Being nervous and jumpy
- Panicking easily
- Being self-conscious and insecure
- Worrying excessively and sometimes obsessively
- Feeling uneasy and trapped with no way out
- Experiencing feelings of doom and gloom
- Feeling that everything is out of control
- Being angry, impatient and irritable
- Being easily wounded by the criticism of others
- Needing to be with others and constantly seeking reassurance
- Feeling isolated and lonely

Physical symptoms include insomnia, hyperactivity, palpitations, rapid and thumping heartbeat (or sometimes a very slow heartbeat), hyperventilation, tightness of the chest, feeling that there is a lump in the throat and difficulty swallowing, gastro-intestinal upset, weakness, tremors, dizziness, a dry mouth, going hot and cold, and sweating.

The fact that anxiety is accompanied by physical symptoms provides strong evidence that it is related to an underlying physiological cause (we examine this in detail in Chapters 3 and 4, pages 40 and 66). The commonest anxiety states are generalised anxiety, often with hypochondria; panic attacks and disorders; and phobias, including agoraphobia. Other less common but more intense conditions include obsessive compulsive disorder (OCD) and post-traumatic stress disorder (PTSD).

Generalised anxiety disorder

It is only human to be anxious about going to the dentist or attending an important meeting; to worry about our children if they are late coming home or about the results of a medical test. If, however, you worry almost constantly and excessively about problems that most people think are minor or events that are unlikely to occur, you may be suffering from generalised anxiety disorder, or GAD. GAD affects about 3 to 4 per cent of the population at any one time in the US and most other Western countries. Women are twice as likely to be affected as men and its onset is generally in childhood.

GAD sufferers worry about virtually everything – on a personal and global scale – and are fearful of the future. They tend to dwell on all the things that can go wrong and are often troubled by constant 'what if?' questions: What if I suffer from cancer? What if I lose my job? Such worries often centre on health, money, family problems and difficulties at work. If you suffer from GAD, the slightest hint that you could have done a task better at work may make you think you're about to be fired; or if your partner says they prefer your hair in another style or don't like the clothes you're wearing, you might see this as a sign of impending separation and divorce. Typically GAD sufferers feel unable to take action or control their thoughts. Jane suffered from intense GAD for several years, in her case specifically because of benzodiazepine withdrawal. Many sufferers try to lead a normal life but others are too seriously affected and are incapable of holding down a job.

GAD is usually diagnosed if your levels of anxiety are so severe that they prevent you functioning normally in your everyday life and persist for more than a few months. Classic symptoms include chronic worry, combined with an inability to turn off such thoughts and relax, feelings of dread and sleeping difficulties. You may also experience physical symptoms that reflect your anxiety but which you interpret as the symptoms of some dread disease. You may overreact, jumping if there is a sudden noise such as a car hooting, or easily become irritable and impatient. The symptoms are likely to be worse at certain times of the day.

If you think you are suffering from GAD it is important that a doctor rule out heart murmurs, diabetes, high blood pressure and an over-active thyroid because, untreated, these conditions can lead to excessive worrying and other health problems. GAD is often poorly diagnosed because it does not have the more intense symptoms that panic attacks and obsessive complusive disorder have. However, there is much that can be done to help sufferers overcome GAD. Certain medications can give relief and talking therapies such as cognitive behavioural therapy are particularly helpful. Breathing control and other biofeedback methods, whereby sufferers learn to control their physical symptoms by sending a signal to the brain that all is well, can also help, as can relaxation techniques. Healthy eating and regular physical exercise are also important in treating this condition successfully.

Panic attacks and panic disorder

Panic attacks are sudden unexpected episodes of intense fear or terror, often accompanied by shortness of breath, rapid pounding heartbeat and choking sensations. Panic disorder is associated with repeated, unexpected panic attacks.

Panic attacks can happen anywhere at any time to some people – they may be out for a stroll or driving and feel perfectly well and happy only to be struck by an attack. Alternatively, panic attacks can occur as part of another mood disorder such as GAD or major depression. They can happen when the sufferer is relaxed – or even asleep, when the attack takes the form of a nightmare so intense that they wake up overwhelmed by fear. Other panic attacks are triggered by specific situations, such as being in certain places or settings.

Symptoms of a panic attack

A full-blown panic attack usually peaks within ten minutes and is associated with some of the following symptoms:

- Shortness of breath or feeling suffocated, with choking sensations

- Palpitations, pounding heart and fast pulse

- Chest pains that can be mistaken for a heart attack

- Sweating, sometimes accompanied by hot and cold flushes

- Gastro-intestinal symptoms such as nausea or diarrhoea

- Dizziness, lightheadedness and fainting; feelings of unreality and a loss of control

Panic attacks are fairly common and it has been estimated that they can affect up to one third of all adults every year in the US, and in the UK at least one person in ten has occasional panic attacks.

If you suffer from frequent panic attacks and have to change your behaviour in order to avoid precipitating an attack you may be diagnosed as suffering from panic disorder. Panic disorder usually develops in the late teens to twenties and is twice as common in women as in men. It rarely begins after the age of 35. It affects about 1.5 per cent of Americans aged 18 to 54 in any given year, while in the UK the incidence of chronic panic disorder is about 2 per cent.[12]

Panic disorder may remain undiagnosed if the doctor simply addresses the physical symptoms reported by the patient. On the other hand, the doctor needs to rule out other physical conditions that can give rise to panic, including minor cardiac problems (if one of the heart valves doesn't close properly – Jane has a mild form of this) or conditions such as irritable bowel syndrome or chronic fatigue syndrome.

If left untreated, panic disorder can lead to depression, substance abuse (if the sufferer self-medicates with drugs or alcohol) and agoraphobia. If you think you have any of the symptoms of panic disorder it is important to discuss them with your doctor. It can be treated successfully with cognitive behavioural therapy and appropriate medication.[13]

Agoraphobia and other phobias

Agoraphobia translates literally as 'fear of the marketplace'. Until recently it was thought to be related to deep-rooted fear of public and open spaces, but it is now considered to be a complication of panic attacks, whereby the sufferer is afraid of having an attack that would be embarrassing or that would occur somewhere where they'd be unable to find help.[14] Most agoraphobics dislike going anywhere unless they are accompanied by someone with whom they feel safe; they may avoid sport and physical exertion for fear of triggering a panic attack or being in areas or situations, such as parties, from where it would be difficult to escape. Agoraphobia affects twice as many women as men.[15]

Cognitive behavioural therapy, which focuses on changing thinking patterns, is particularly effective in dealing with agoraphobia.[16] Understanding what is actually happening to the body – simply that the so-called 'fight or flight' response has been triggered – is also very helpful (this is examined in detail in Chapter 3). Biofeedback techniques are valuable in controlling these disorders, as is controlled exposure to the situations that trigger panic in you. Cognitive behavioural therapy may also be used to induce some of the sensations experienced during panic, such as fast heartbeat, in order to train you that a fast heartbeat is something you need not fear. A similar technique of progressive controlled exposure is used to treat other specific phobias which can trigger panic, such as fear of snakes or dogs. Learning relaxation techniques such as meditation (discussed further in Chapters 7 and 9) can help with all panic conditions. Well-known agoraphobics include Woody Allen, Kim Basinger and the late Roy Castle.

Obsessive compulsive disorder

Obsessive compulsive disorder, or OCD, is a particularly unpleasant type of chronic anxiety disorder whereby sufferers often feel that they have lost control and that their brain is forcing them to think the same thoughts or do the same senseless things over and over again. If you suffer from OCD you are likely to be troubled by recurrent and intrusive thoughts (obsessions) and by compulsions to carry out repeatedly certain physical tasks, such as hand washing or hoarding things, and mental acts such as repeatedly counting the same sequence of numbers. Obsessions often centre on dirt, germs and disease or fear of behaving badly. People with OCD usually want to please others and are often especially anxious socially, but they often feel they must avoid other people, especially in situations that might involve stimuli that induce their condition.

The illness usually starts in adolescence or sometimes early childhood and, unlike most other mood disorders, it affects males and females equally. Old psychodynamic theories of OCD, which viewed it as repressed anger or a need to try to control the environment which felt inherently uncontrollable, have been replaced by new evidence, based on brain imaging, which shows that it is related to overactivity of one or more parts and circuits in the brain. The problem is thought to lie in the circuit that links the caudate nucleus in the limbic system with the frontal lobes in the cerebrum, where thinking and planning take place. This normally prompts you to wash or to remember your keys, for example. The caudate nucleus has close links with the amygdala, or fear centre, which is now thought to be the source of the problem of OCD – which explains why sufferers experience such intense anxiety. (On page 61 we look in more detail at the role of the amygdala in triggering anxiety and depression.) Recent studies using MRI scans suggest that OCD sufferers also have reduced amounts of grey matter in the parts of the brain important in suppressing habits.[17]

The suggestion that OCD relates to an underlying physiological problem with the brain dates back to the recognition in the 1920s that its onset could follow trauma to the brain and encephalitis. Indeed, many doctors now regard OCD as a neurological disease[18] but as we shall argue later in the book, many mood disorders might be viewed in a similar light if a more scientific approach were used to study and diagnose them. There is much that can be done to treat OCD – there is strong evidence, for example, that some talking therapies are effective in dealing with OCD, as are a number of other approaches (see Chapter 7, pages 131–48).

Post-traumatic stress disorder (PTSD)

Post-traumatic stress disorder, or PTSD, is a debilitating mental condition that is caused by a deeply disturbing experience or a prolonged series of such events. The symptoms have been recognised for centuries – over which time it has been given various names, the best known being shell shock – but it was defined only in 1980, based on the experiences of soldiers and victims of the Vietnam War. It is often associated with service personnel who have undergone the trauma of combat[19] but it can affect anyone who has been involved in, or witnessed, events that provoked intense fear, helplessness or horror.

PTSD produces various unwanted emotional responses and can emerge weeks, months or years after the event. Often the events are re-experienced through intrusive memories, nightmares, hallucinations or flashbacks, usually triggered by anything that symbolises or resembles the trauma. Troubled sleep, irritability, anger, poor concentration, hypervigilance and exaggerated responses are common symptoms. Sufferers may feel depression, detachment or estrangement, guilt, intense anxiety and panic, and other negative emotions. On their return from active service, soldiers with PTSD often experience an acute sense of having little in common with civilian peers.

There is greater recognition of the mental health consequences of traumatic experiences now and much research has been done in the past 25 years. An effective new method of treating PTSD is discussed on pages 151–7.

Depression

Depression is increasingly common and is often associated with anxiety, especially in women. It is a particularly cruel condition in which the sufferer experiences intense feelings of hopelessness, an almost total lack of self-esteem and an inability to concentrate or make decisions. Usually there is a marked lack of interest in pleasure or activity and sufferers often appear totally self-obsessed because their minds, and too often their conversation, keep returning to the same hurts, anxieties and sorrows. Indeed Jane's mother, in referring to her father's depression, called it 'the selfishness disease', because that is how it appeared to her. Sadly, this is how depression often appears to partners, family and friends and this perceived self-absorption tends to make people draw back just when the sufferer desperately needs the help and support of others. This is partly why depression can destroy family and work relationships and friendships.

Clinical depression, so-called because it is disabling, now affects about 2 to 3 per cent of the UK population at any one time and about 5 per cent of the population of the USA, where a staggering 17 per cent of people experience a major episode at some time in their lives.[20] Many sufferers do not seek treatment, partly because of fear of stigmatisation. Untreated depression is the leading cause of suicide.

The main symptoms of depression

- Feeling unhappy most of the time

- Loss of interest in life and failure to enjoy anything

- Difficulty in making decisions

- Inability to cope

- Tiredness and fatigue

- Change of appetite and weight

- Disturbed sleep with early-morning waking

- Problems with memory

- Time appearing to pass very slowly

- Loss of self-confidence

- Feeling useless, inadequate and hopeless

- Withdrawal from social contact

- Feeling worse at particular times of the day, usually in the morning

- Loss of interest in sex

- Thoughts of suicide (especially in major or endogenous depression or breakdown)

Note: the exact symptoms experienced and their intensity vary widely, depending on the severity of the depression.

There are a number of different types of depression, although with the exception of some specific conditions, such as seasonal affective disorder and post-natal depression, classification is controversial. Indeed some types of depression such as atypical depression or dysthymic depression are poorly understood. In part, this is due to the fact that conventional diagnosis is based on symptoms reported by the sufferer rather than the results of medical tests. It is likely that the symptoms of heart disease would be equally confused if there were no scans and medical diagnostic tests and diagnosis were based simply on the patient's description of their symptoms.

Some international scientists now base their classification – and treatment – of the different types of depression on imbalances in different groups of neurotransmitters or on the result of functional brain scans.[21] This is a far more scientific approach that lends itself to accurate diagnosis and improved treatment (this approach is examined in

Chapter 5), but unfortunately it has yet to be widely adopted. Let us look at some of the types of depression distinguished by Western psychiatry on the basis of reported symptoms, as these are the classifications you may hear your doctor or other health professionals use. Some, such as atypical depression, are particularly poorly defined.

Major depression

Major depression used to be called endogenous (from within) depression because it was believed that there was no apparent cause for the illness. It was considered more likely to reflect a genetic component than reactive depression, which was thought to be triggered by a stressful event. The distinction between endogenous and reactive depression is no longer thought to apply and both types are regarded as major depression, depending on the severity of the symptoms (see box above). The relationship between major depression and stress and other risk factors is discussed in Chapter 4, and diagnostic methods of clearly distinguishing major depression from other types of depression are described in Chapter 5.

In serious cases, major depression can turn into total mental exhaustion, which used to be called a nervous breakdown. Interestingly, this is equivalent to what is known as behavioural despair in animals (see page 65).

Dysthymic depression

Dysthymic depression is usually diagnosed by Western medicine on the basis of the severity and number of symptoms and the duration of the illness. It is considered to be a mild form of depression that lasts for a period of no less than two years. A diagnosis of dysthymia rather than major depressive illness is usually made because there are not enough symptoms present to fulfil the diagnostic criteria for major depression or the symptoms may come and go for a few days at a time. Because dysthymia is chronic it is often many years before the sufferer seeks help. However, if the condition is not addressed it can worsen or the sufferer may experience serious illness known as double depression and in some cases breakdown. Dysthymia is thought to affect about 10.9 million American adults, about 1.6 per cent of the population.[22] In Canada, 3–6 per cent of adults will get dysthymia during their lifetime.[23]

Dysthymia is known to respond differently to treatment than major depression. Commonly prescribed antidepressants may not work and it can take months to find an effective treatment. Better diagnosis and treatment of dysthymic depression is discussed in Chapter 5.

Atypical depression

Atypical depression (AD) is a subtype of depression characterised by being able to experience improved mood in response to positive events.[24] In contrast, sufferers of 'melancholic' depression generally cannot experience positive moods, even when good things happen. Additionally, atypical depression is characterised by over-eating and over-sleeping rather than the loss of appetite and insomnia that characterise most other types of depression. There is sometimes a heavy leaden feelings in the limbs. One of the most characteristic features of this type of depression is that it is responsive to treatment with SSRI and MAO antidepressants but not tricyclic antidepressants, although the reasons for this are not understood (see pages 116–19).

Despite its name, 'atypical' depression is actually the most common subtype of depression, affecting up to 40 per cent of those suffering from depression generally.[25]

Bipolar disorder (manic depression)

Bipolar disorder – often referred to as manic depression – is characterised by periods of depression interspersed with periods of mania. During the depressive phase sufferers will experience symptoms similar to those outlined in the box on page 33, while in the manic phase they often have boundless energy, very high self-esteem and little need for sleep. They may also act impulsively or even recklessly and be driven to take excessive risks, for example in sexual or business situations.

There are several suggestions as to the cause of bipolar disorder, including high or low levels of neurotransmitters or imbalances between them or a change in sensitivity of nerve cell receptors. Treatment frequently involves medication, most commonly lithium. This is a natural mineral and its use was for many years opposed by conventional medicine. Some scientists believe that lithium deficiency can cause a range of mental illnesses and in Chapter 10 you'll find guidance on ensuring an adequate intake in the diet.

Bipolar disorder can be difficult to diagnose and symptoms may be masked, especially if the sufferer has attempted to self-medicate with alcohol or drugs. In some cases bipolar disorder and schizophrenia may be diagnosed in the same patient by different psychiatrists.[26]

Seasonal Affective Disorder

Seasonal affective disorder, or SAD, is a type of clinical depression that occurs in a small percentage of people, especially women, living at high latitudes in either the northern or southern hemisphere. In Britain it is thought to affect about one person in 50.[27] The condition is extremely rare in those living within 30 degrees of the Equator. Symptoms often begin when the sufferer is in their twenties or thirties, and they usually recur regularly each winter, starting between September and November in the northern hemisphere and continuing until March or April. Symptoms tend to be more physical than psychological and are thought to reflect physiological responses to the environment rather than being triggered by emotional pain. They commonly include fatigue and the need to sleep for longer, cravings for carbohydrates and sweet foods, and marked mood swings. The disorder was not recognised until the 1980s when researchers at the National Institute of Mental Health in the USA developed diagnostic criteria for what had previously been called 'winter depression'.[28]

The precise problem that a lack of light causes in affected individuals is not known, but it is thought to involve cortisol and thyroid hormones and to be associated with decreased levels of neurotransmitters such as serotonin. Recent evidence suggests that it is associated with a problem with the diurnal pattern of melatonin secretion which begins earlier in the evenings and lasts longer in the mornings in SAD sufferers.[29] Some scientists equate SAD with hibernating behaviour and suggest it is entirely normal in certain people. Most of us feel much better mentally and emotionally during long sunny days, and light therapy can help not only sufferers of SAD but also many other conditions, as you will discover in Chapter 8. In Hippocrates' day, sufferers from what is thought to have been SAD were told to look at the sun – but we certainly do not recommend this!

Post-natal depression

Post-natal depression is a particularly distressing condition that affects about one in ten mothers. It usually develops four to six weeks after childbirth, although it can occur several months later. Its exact cause is not known but it is thought there are a number of contributing factors, including a history of depression, either personally or a family history; experiencing stressful events during pregnancy or a prolonged or difficult labour; problems with the baby's health; and a lack or perceived lack of support for the mother.[30]

The symptoms of post-natal depression are similar to those of depression generally (see box on page 33), although sufferers are particularly prone to worrying that they are not enjoying their new baby as they feel they should; feeling 'edgy' and irritable; disturbed sleep, even when the baby is quiet; and feeling worthless and unable to cope. Anxiety about all manner of things is also common, as are thoughts of suicide.

If you suspect you may be suffering from post-natal depression it is vital that you get help. Post-natal depression can be a particularly important factor in maintaining intergenerational problems of anxiety and depression, so finding help is important for the baby's sake as well as your own.[31] Thankfully, there is much that can be done to prevent and treat post-natal depression, for example good nutrition, appropriate support and help for new mothers, and breast-feeding can all help (see page 71).

Post-natal psychosis

Post-natal psychosis is an uncommon but severe form of post-natal depression. It affects between one and three in 1,000 new mothers in the UK. Mothers who have previously suffered from a serious mental illness – or who have a family history of serious mental illness – are the most prone to it. In addition to the symptoms of severe depression, post-natal psychosis is characterised by delusions, hallucinations (such as hearing voices), odd behaviour and irrational thoughts. Both the mother's and baby's lives can be at risk and early treatment is crucial.

WHAT TO DO

If you think you may be suffering from any of the illnesses outlined in this chapter, the first thing to do is to seek help from your local doctor and obtain an accurate diagnosis of your condition. We urge you not to miss the next two chapters, which outline what is going on in the brain in mood disorders and the risk factors involved, but if you are feeling particularly unwell and desperate at the moment you may find it useful to read Chapter 5, which gives advice on obtaining the best help, support and treatment available from public and private healthcare systems. Many new treatments are becoming available for those suffering from anxiety and depression, so the outlook is much brighter than it was 20 years ago. Furthermore, many of the conditions outlined in this chapter respond to improved diet and lifestyle and it is not always necessary to use drug treatments.

Chapter Three

Mind Matters

WHEN WE TELL PEOPLE that we have suffered from mental illness they generally look shocked and surprised. Perhaps this is because we appear to be well-presented 'together' people, carrying out professional work, so we don't fit the stereotype of the mentally ill. Or perhaps they're surprised that we're willing to talk openly about mental illness – something that many people still regard as shameful or, at the very least, embarrassing. It's important, therefore, to emphasise again that mental illness is not an indication that a person is weak or flawed.

The fears that are at the root of negative, unhelpful attitudes to mental illness stem from a basic lack of understanding of the brain–mind–body system and what can go wrong to cause mental illnesses such as anxiety and depression. In order to understand why these mood disorders are so common, and can be so difficult to treat using orthodox drug-based medicine alone, you need to acquire some basic knowledge about the brain–mind–body system and its workings.

If you are tempted to skip this chapter, again we ask you not to – if you understand something of the root causes of mental illness, you are in a powerful position to choose the most effective treatment if you or your loved ones are ever affected. Remember our experiences, recounted in Chapter 1: in both cases our symptoms were seriously misdiagnosed and the wrong medication prescribed. It would have helped a great deal if we and our families had had a better understanding of our conditions and been able to play a more prominent role in discussing treatments and outcomes with the health professionals involved.

Hopefully, you will also find that developing a rational understanding of the problems of mental illness will help to dispel any frightening images and unfounded fears that you may have. According to the distinguished medical journalist Rita Carter in *Mapping the Mind*, the latest scanning and imaging techniques, which show three-dimensional images of the brain and highlight areas of brain activity, mean that, 'The biological basis of mental illness is now demonstrable: no one can reasonably watch the frenzied, localised activity in the brain of a person driven by some obsession, or see the dull glow of a depressed brain and doubt that these are physical conditions rather than some ineffable sickness of the soul.'[1] Recognising that anxiety and depression reflect real physiological problems in the brain, rather than being frightening abstract afflictions or character flaws, provides a much better basis for assessing effective methods of prevention and treatment.

Don't be put off by jargon

Many of the words used to describe the brain and its functions are derived from Greek or Latin, once the international languages of scholars. This can be off-putting so we've tried to avoid jargon as much as possible, although some is unavoidable. It's unfortunate that this outdated scientific jargon has not been translated into English to make it more accessible. Perhaps this is because talking about the locus (place) coeruleus (blue) sounds so much more impressive than talking about the blue area of the brain! The first time we use such words they are explained.

The chapter is in three parts: first we discuss the components of the brain–mind–body system by comparing it with a modern computer; then we describe how it works – for example, how messages or feelings are transmitted; finally we describe what goes wrong with the system when we are stressed, anxious or depressed.

THE BRAIN–MIND–BODY SYSTEM

Until fairly recently, Western thinking about the brain was dominated by the ideas of the seventeenth-century French philosopher and scientist René Descartes, who argued that the brain, mind and body are each separate entities. This led to a highly simplistic view of illness, especially mental illness, as something that can be isolated and treated physically or chemically, with drugs. We now know this to be entirely wrong and that the brain (physical structure, cells and chemicals), mind (thoughts, ideas, feelings and images) and body are inextricably linked. For example, in response to stress, the body releases hormones that can depress the immune system, leaving the body more prone to ill health. You may have noticed that if you have a stressful event in your life you may become ill. These stress hormones also enter the brain, causing it to increase levels of some key chemical messengers (neurotransmitters) which can eventually become depleted, leading to anxiety and depression.

Our amazing biochemical computer

The brain can be regarded as an amazingly complex biochemical computer, controlling the brain–mind–body system through a maze of nerves and chemical messengers. It enables us constantly to adjust and readjust to our changing physical, social and emotional environment and to maintain homeostasis, the internal metabolic equilibrium that is essential to our survival.

The human brain is, of course, immeasurably more sophisticated than any computer. Indeed it is the most complex object in the known universe. All day, every day it takes in signals from our surroundings – the things we see and hear, touch, smell and feel – and attempts to process and integrate them so that we adapt and maintain control of ourselves and our lives. The brain is affected by everything that happens to us: our experiences, actions and thoughts; illnesses and infections; as well as chemicals circulating in the bloodstream and chemicals produced by the brain itself. In addition to processing information and making decisions, the brain can cause us to experience happiness and pleasure or pain and distress.

Let's look at how the brain functions when it is performing well, before considering some of the latest surprising findings on the root causes of anxiety and depression.

Mission control

The brain is a grey mass weighing about 1.5 kg (3 lb). It is roughly the size of a coconut and is shaped rather like a large walnut with deep wrinkles in it. Although there are significant differences between the right and left sides of the brain, it is, like much of the rest of the human body, roughly symmetrical. With the exception of the tiny pineal gland at the base of the brain, every module is duplicated between the two hemispheres. For simplicity, we refer to only one module throughout. Some of the most important structures of the brain are shown overleaf.

Many of us remember from our school biology lessons that the brain is connected to the rest of the body through the spinal cord and stringy nerves known as the peripheral nervous system which, for example, signals the body to move. As well as being linked to the rest of the body physically, however, the brain also controls the body chemically, because it is connected through the hypothalamus directly to the master gland of the hormone system, the pituitary gland. Hence it can send powerful chemical messages, including surges of hormones through the body. Surges of adrenaline, for example, equip the body for 'fight or flight'. It is these chemicals that cause some of the most unpleasant physical symptoms of anxiety and depression such as rapid or irregular heartbeats. The brain is also linked to the immune system through a system of chemicals known as cytokines.

These three integrated systems – the nervous, endocrine (hormone)

The brain

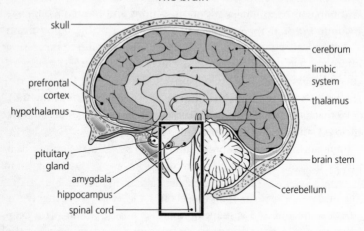

skull
cerebrum
limbic system
prefrontal cortex
thalamus
hypothalamus
pituitary gland
amygdala
hippocampus
spinal cord
brain stem
cerebellum

Centres for neurotransmitter production in the brain stem, enlarged

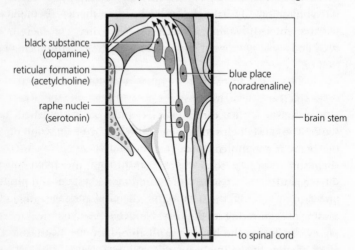

black substance (dopamine)
reticular formation (acetylcholine)
raphe nuclei (serotonin)
blue place (noradrenaline)
brain stem
to spinal cord

The human brain is shown in dark grey, the old mammalian brain in paler grey, and the reptilian brain in white.

and immune systems – are the principal guardians of the brain–mind–body system. Our ability to adapt to changing environments so as to maintain equilibrium depends on these three systems and the brain's ability to integrate them effectively.

Defending the territory

The brain is so important that, unlike other organs such as the liver or stomach or even the heart, it has special protection and is entirely enclosed within a bony helmet called the skull. Within the skull the brain floats in the cerebrospinal fluid, which helps to absorb physical shocks thus minimising any potential damage to the brain from external sources. The cerebrospinal fluid also transfers nutrients to the cells and removes waste from them.

As well as having this strong physical protection, the brain, its blood vessels and the cerebrospinal fluid in which it floats are protected from viruses and chemicals circulating in the main bloodstream by the blood–brain barrier. This is not a simple physical barrier. It is a physiological barrier that reflects the fact that all the blood vessels that enter the brain are much less leaky than elsewhere in the body and also have special linings and 'wrappings' (comprising fatty glial cells).

The blood–brain barrier is permeable to water, oxygen and glucose, which are the brain's main fuels, as well as to the waste products of metabolism, such as carbon dioxide, and to small fat-soluble molecules. The barrier helps to keep out unwanted chemicals and protect the brain from unpredictable (but normal) fluctuations in blood chemistry. However, some psychoactive chemicals, including fat-soluble pesticides and other pollutants and recreational and prescription drugs, can cross the barrier and reach the brain, in some cases causing or aggravating stress, anxiety and depression. There is increasing evidence that the blood–brain barrier becomes permeable as a result of stress (including heat stress),[2] illness[3] and chemicals.[4]

The blood–brain barrier

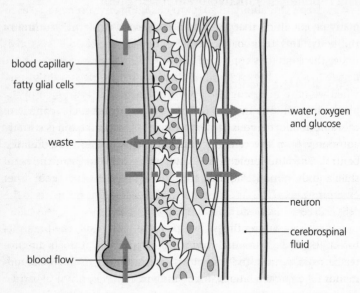

blood capillary

fatty glial cells

water, oxygen and glucose

waste

neuron

cerebrospinal fluid

blood flow

From animal to human

The human brain actually comprises three brains which evolved in three key stages of our evolution from reptiles to mammals to humans. The reptilian brain, or brain stem, is concerned with our basic survival and developed first during the dinosaur era. It was followed about 100 million years later by the development of the emotional brain (often referred to as the old mammalian brain) or limbic system, which has the capacity for emotions such as happiness, disgust or fear and also has a system for storing memories. The third very recent phase of evolution resulted in the cerebrum, or cerebral cortex. Sometimes called the 'human' brain, the cerebrum is capable of logical abstract thought, the use of language and numbers, problem-solving and creativity.

According to the famous American neuroscientist Paul Maclean, the three brains within us can be thought of as three biological computers which, although interconnected, each retain their special types of intelligence, subjectivity, sense of time and space, memory, mobility and other less specific functions.[5]

The reptilian, instinctive brain (brain stem)

Many people think that the conscious brain is entirely in control of the body. This is probably because the skeletomuscular system is under the conscious control of the cerebrum. So, for example, if we decide to sit up, walk around or clasp our hands, we can do so provided we have no serious illness or incapacity. In fact, much of the body, especially the internal visceral organs, is under the control of the autonomic nervous system which, as its name suggests, has autonomy from the cerebral cortex and hence from our conscious control. The autonomic nervous system operates through the brain stem and the hypothalamus in the limbic system to control our inner environment.

The brain stem is the oldest, most primitive part of the brain, inherited from our reptilian ancestors. It is a relatively simple structure at the top of the spinal cord and is responsible for the instinctive reactions essential for self-preservation, including reflexes and commands for approach, attack, flight and mating.

Importantly, the brain stem is also in control of our unconscious basic life functions such as breathing, heartbeat and the fight-or-flight response. Because these functions are under the control of the autonomic nervous system, we cannot, for example, instruct our hearts to beat more slowly or tell our digestive systems how quickly or slowly to process our food. This point is important, because many scientists now consider anxiety and depression to be disorders of the autonomic nervous system (see page 59).

The cerebellum

The cerebellum is one of the most evolutionarily primitive brain regions and looks similar in fish, reptiles, birds and mammals, suggesting that it performs similar essential functions in all vertebrate species. It plays an important role in integrating sensory perceptions and movement.

The switch between primitive instinct and rational thought

Human evolution means that some of the functions of the instinctive, reptilian brain can now be controlled by the intellectual, analytical cerebrum. For example, most of us don't physically attack people who have made us angry. Nevertheless, when primitive instincts generated by fear or anger dominate our actions it is because the reptilian brain is overriding the cerebrum. This occurs because an 'arousal' switch in the brain stem has been turned on, which effectively shuts down the logical brain allowing instinct to take over, causing us to react immediately. It switches off again once the threat is removed, but in the meantime we are likely to suffer acute stress as a result of the reaction we experience.

Moreover, although self-awareness is associated with the cerebrum, it is the brain stem that is critical for maintaining alertness and the sleep–awake cycle which can be so disrupted in anxiety and depression. This part of the brain is active even when we are deeply asleep. It is also from the brain stem that many of the important neurotransmitters that affect our mood are distributed to other areas of the brain (see diagram on page 44).

The old mammalian emotional brain (limbic system)

The emotional brain (the limbic system) is dominated by appetites and urges, pleasant and unpleasant feelings, playful behaviour and emotions for nurturing and protecting the young. It began to evolve millions of years later than the reptilian brain and is superimposed on it. The hypothalamus in the limbic system is connected to the pituitary gland, which releases chemical messengers known as hormones. These can give rise to the physical expressions of our emotions. We can, for example, go hot and cold in response to a sudden shock, or the heart can start to beat very fast if something suddenly frightens us.

The centre for long-term explicit memory, the hippocampus, and the centre for emotional implicit memory, the amygdala, are also located in the limbic system (see page 50). The hippocampus helps us to remember day-to-day events and to find our way around: London taxi drivers, for example, have been found to have extra-large hippocampuses. The amygdala, on the other hand, is where our awareness of danger is centred. It is essential for self-preservation as it generates and registers fear and stores powerful emotional memories. The amgydala is now thought by scientists to be central to the development of many types of anxiety and depressive illnesses. When triggered, it can make us feel frightened and anxious and it can generate fight-or-flight reactions through the autonomic nervous system by causing stress hormones such as adrenaline and cortisol to be released.

The limbic system has a much simpler structure than the cerebrum and is able to process information much faster – to equip us to react rapidly to danger. Dr David Servan-Schreiber, Professor of Psychiatry at the University of Pittsburgh and author of *Healing without Freud or Prozac*, illustrates the different roles of the emotional brain and the cerebrum with the example of how each would react to a piece of wood that resembled a snake: the older brain sets off a reaction of fear based on partial and erroneous information before the cerebrum has even begun to determine that the object is harmless.[6]

The human, logical brain (cerebrum)

Our third brain, the cerebrum, is the rational, analytical brain. Modern humans belong to the species *Homo sapiens*, meaning wise or intelligent man, a species that evolved only 200,000 years ago. It is this brain that defines our humanity.

The cerebrum is concerned with visual processing, sound and speech, and with aspects of memory, orientation, calculation and pattern recognition. It also integrates functions such as thinking, analysing, conceptualising and planning. The highly complex network of neural cells that make up the cerebrum enabled humans to develop language as a basis for intellectual tasks such as reading and writing, to understand mathematical calculation and to generate ideas and concepts. It also plays a major role in our conscious appreciation of emotion, and in registering and communicating feelings emanating from the unconscious mind, including those related to anxiety and depression. Feelings are generated in the emotional, instinctive older brains, but it is the cerebrum that articulates them and can help us to gain control over them.

One particularly advanced part of the cerebrum, the prefrontal cortex, appears to be strongly affected by anxiety and depression. It is situated in the frontal lobes of the cerebrum (see diagram page 44) and has many connections with the limbic system and the brain stem – the older, deeper brain structures. The many connections between the prefrontal cortex, where the working memory is centred, and the amygdala, the centre of the implicit emotional memory, have been confirmed by functional magnetic resonance imaging (MRI) studies in laboratory animals and humans.[7]

One of the main functions of the prefrontal cortex is the control of pleasure, pain, anger, rage, panic and the emotional mind. It helps suppress urges that could lead to socially unacceptable behaviour. However, sudden threats and stress can temporarily disable the prefrontal cortex, allowing the brain to react without thinking. In the last few decades, brain-imaging studies have indicated that the volume of the prefrontal cortex and the number of its interconnections with other regions of the brain are reduced in people subjected to chronic or recurring stress and in those with chronic depression. Other studies show that it can be regenerated, however, once the depression has been treated successfully.[8]

Time for reflection

It is worth taking a moment to consider what the evolution of the brain means for human biology. The Earth is 4,500 million years old, but it is difficult for most of us to appreciate this enormous period of time. If we convert this period to a single 24 hour day, then the reptilian brain began to evolve at about 22.20 hours but amazingly the cerebrum evolved at only a fraction of a second before midnight.

Three brains in one – the conscious and unconscious mind

A useful way to think of the three brains within us is to consider the differing characteristics of snakes, dogs and human beings. Snakes are entirely instinctive, completely lacking in emotion and concerned only with survival and breeding. In contrast, dogs are instinctive but they are also loving, nurturing, emotional creatures. Human beings have all the characteristics of snakes and dogs but, in addition, are capable of analysis, creative and logical thinking and great intellectual achievement.

As Freud observed, it is the unconscious mind, which we now know to be in the reptilian and old mammalian brain, where much of our turmoil takes place – although it is registered, verbalised and communicated by the cerebrum, the conscious mind. The importance of the interrelationship between the two old brains and the cerebrum explains the use of frontal lobotomy, which was once a standard treatment for almost all types of mental illness. The aim of the operation was to sever the link between the unconscious mind (the reptilian and emotional brains), where emotions are generated, from the cerebrum, where they are registered by the conscious mind, by cutting through the nerve fibres that connected them. (Chapter 8 looks at the use of this procedure, and its history is discussed briefly in Chapter 11.) Thankfully there are now many less drastic means of helping the cerebrum take control over our older, more unruly brains.

HOW THE BRAIN–MIND–BODY SYSTEM WORKS

Transmitting nervous energy

The brain is an amazingly clever electrochemical system. It works by moving around tiny chemical particles (called ions) which have positive electrical charges to turn on its circuits, or ions with negative charges to turn off its circuits (see diagram page 54). These electrical circuits are controlled by vitally important chemicals known as neurotransmitters (which work at a local level, unlike neurohormones which act as chemical messengers to distant parts of the brain). Thickly insulated nerves transmit signals between the brain and the rest of the body – just like electric wires in your house.

The fat controller

The electrical insulation of the brain and nervous system is provided by fat, which forms myelin sheaths to protect nerves – see diagram page 54. Just as we used to use rubber, and now use plastics, to insulate the wires that carry electrical currents along particular pathways in electrical devices, so the brain uses fats. It is therefore a very fatty organ, containing 60 per cent fats (compared with less than 20 per cent in other organs). Many scientists and doctors now think that the Western diet, which is full of bad fats and deficient in good fats, is an important cause of depression. (For further information on this see Chapter 10.)

Rivers of the mind

A single nerve consists of hundreds of thousands of neurons, the tiny cells that create brain activity. The billions of neurons in the human brain transmit the electrochemical signals communicating, cell to cell, along pathways from and to the brain. Many of these begin in the reptilian brain.

Interestingly, the brain can constantly learn and reprogramme itself. It does this not by altering neurons but by building or strengthening the connections between them, effectively rewiring itself. This theory was first proposed by the great Spanish neuroscientist Ramon y Cajal in 1894, but it was not demonstrated experimentally until towards the end of the twentieth century when Nobel prizewinning neuroscientist Eric Kandel carried out his classic studies. According to Kandel the process of rewiring occurs because genes, as well as shaping our bodies, constantly alter our brains as we respond to experience.[9]

A neuron has three main parts (see diagram page 54): the cell body, which contains the nucleus; the axon, the extension of the neuron that transmits messages to other neurons; and dendrites, extensions of neurons which receive messages from other cells. Because neurons don't actually touch, there is a tiny, fluid-filled gap, known as a synapse, between the transmitting axon of one neuron and the receiving dendrite of the other. It is the reconfiguring of synapses that helps the brain to adapt to experiences and the environment: 'you are your synapses', as Joseph Le Doux has said.[9]

Jumping the gap

In order for an electrical charge, the nerve impulse, to be transmitted, it must cross this gap, just like the spark in the sparking plug of a car engine. Neurotransmitters, released from the axon of the transmitting neuron, cross the synapse, attach to receptors on the receiving dendrite and effectively unlock gates that enable ions to move into the receiving neuron and pass on the electrical signal. Neurotransmitters that increase the activity of neurons are called excitory, while those that calm them down are called inhibitory. Some neurotransmitters, such as dopamine, can increase or decrease the signal according to the type of receptor they bind to. The entire nervous system is a balance between excitory or stimulatory forces and inhibitory forces.

Neurotransmitters: the brain's chemical messengers

Many doctors and psychiatrists now believe that the key to understanding mental illness lies in understanding neurotransmitters. While this can lead to an oversimplification of the complexities of mental illness, there is no doubt that levels of neurotransmitters in the brain are crucial to mental health. Put simply, when levels of important neurotransmitters become depleted or unbalanced the brain's circuits don't work properly. Moreover, neurotransmitters play a key role in creating new connections in the brain, helping it to rewire itself.[9] Many of the drugs used to treat mood disorders are designed to increase the action of neurotransmitters on receptors or the levels of neurotransmitters at synapses. The fact that neurotransmitters help the brain rewire itself may explain why drugs aimed at correcting deficiencies in serotonin or noradrenaline can take several weeks to work.

Communication between neurons

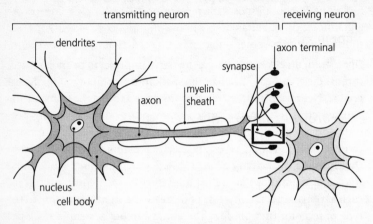

transmitting neuron

receiving neuron

dendrites

axon terminal

synapse

axon

myelin
sheath

nucleus

cell body

a synapse, enlarged

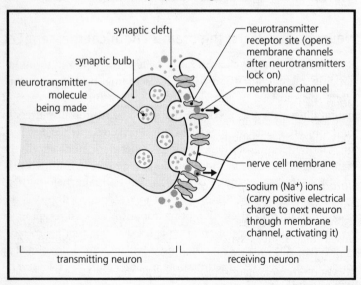

synaptic cleft

neurotransmitter
receptor site (opens
membrane channels
after neurotransmitters
lock on)

synaptic bulb

neurotransmitter
molecule
being made

membrane channel

nerve cell membrane

sodium (Na$^+$) ions
(carry positive electrical
charge to next neuron
through membrane
channel, activating it)

transmitting neuron

receiving neuron

Some important neurotransmitters

The brain has many different neurotransmitters to fulfil its complex functions. For our purposes the most important neurotransmitters are glutamic acid (or glutamate); gamma-aminobutyric acid (GABA for short); the monoamines – dopamine, noradrenaline and serotonin; and the endorphins.

Neurotransmitters and diet

Most neurotransmitters are manufactured in the brain from precursor substances. They are therefore called 'non-essential' since they do not need to be taken in as part of the diet. However, certain elements in the diet are essential for making neurotransmitters, and nutrition is increasingly seen as being important in maintaining mental health (see Chapter 10).

Workhorse neurotransmitters

Glutamate and GABA are the main workhorse neurotransmitters. They are widely distributed throughout the brain and occur at relatively high concentrations. They form a pair, whereby glutamate is always excitory and GABA is always inhibitory.

Glutamate, the get-up-and-go neurotransmitter

One of glutamate's vital functions is in learning and the laying down of long-term memories. Some neurotoxins such as mercury, which caused 'mad hatter's syndrome', cause high levels of glutamate to build up in the brain, which leads to agitation. Foods with added monosodium glutamate (MSG), including many Japanese and Chinese foods, have also been linked to agitation (see pages 217). Some of the latest drugs to treat depression target glutamate (see pages 116–17 for more details).

GABA, the tranquillity neurotransmitter

GABA is the principal inhibitory neurotransmitter of the brain. GABA receptors increase tranquillity by inhibiting neuronal activity. It is present in 30 to 40 per cent of all synapses and its concentration in the brain is 200 to 1,000 times that of monoamines such as serotonin. It is particularly concentrated in the parts of the brain concerned with the unconscious mind (the brain stem and limbic system).

Substances that enhance the effect of GABA on receptors are often used to counteract anxiety, the most frequently diagnosed psychiatric disorder throughout the Western world. In the past, benzodiazepines were the most frequently prescribed drugs for anxiety; alcohol and barbiturates have similar effects on the GABA receptors. One of the principal effects of alcohol is to shut down circuits in the brain, producing a major inhibitory effect in the higher cerebral centres concerned with inhibition and judgement, especially the prefrontal cortex, as well as the parts of the limbic system that affect co-ordination and movement.

Monoamine neurotransmitters

The monoamines, so-called because of their chemical structure, occur at much lower concentrations than the workhorse neurotransmitters. However, they are involved in emotion and mood, as well as motivation, sleep and appetite, and adequate levels are crucial for achieving a balanced and motivated outlook and a healthy appetite and sleep pattern. The monoamines are secreted by centres in the brain stem (see diagram page 44).

Dopamine, the arousal neurotransmitter

Dopamine is vital for physical motivation and it controls arousal in many parts of the brain, including those important in appetite, eating, pleasure and sex. Higher levels of dopamine in the brain have been linked to creativity and the ability to visualise and to formulate 'what if?' questions.

The brain has a 'reward circuit' in which dopamine is the main neurotransmitter. The purpose of this is to encourage activities that are good for us individually and for the survival of the species, such as eating good food and taking part in sexual activity. However, the process can be subverted by the use of drugs. The role of dopamine in generating intense pleasure in the brain, by activating its reward circuit, is now thought to be crucial to understanding most types of addiction. One of the principal effects of cocaine, for example, is to increase dopamine levels in synapses in the brain's reward circuit. As a result, long-term users can lose the ability to experience any normal pleasure because of neuron degeneration (burn out) from over-production of dopamine. General dopamine depletion throughout the brain contributes to a particularly severe type of depression which commonly results from drug abuse.

Chocolate and falling in love

Phenylethylamine, a chemical found in chocolate, has a similar structure to amphetamine and is thought to cause both dopamine and endorphin release. It is the chemical that is released in the brain when animals bond or, in human terms, fall in love. Its highest concentration is in part of the brain's reward circuit. This could explain why chocolate is associated with love and excitement.

Noradrenaline, the attention neurotransmitter

Noradrenaline, also known as norepinephrine, is most active when we are awake and appears to play a role in focusing attention, fixing information in the long-term memory and helping to establish new memories.

Importantly, it is the main neurotransmitter of the sympathetic nervous system which controls the fight-or-flight reaction, changing our physiology and increasing the heart rate and blood pressure (see pages 59–61). Noradrenaline is found throughout the brain, but only in a tiny percentage of the brain's synapses. More than half the brain's noradrenaline is concentrated in two small areas, both of which are associated with the brain's alarm system: the amygdala and the locus coeruleus, or blue place, the centre of anxiety but also a pleasure centre in the brain stem (see diagram page 44). Noradrenaline is released during panic attacks and when we experience stress or an anxiety state. Beta-blocking medication, originally used to treat heart conditions and now frequently used to treat stress and anxiety, works by blocking the activity of noradrenaline.

Noradrenaline levels are also high relative to serotonin in some types of depression: conversely some types of depression are associated with noradrenaline deficiency and are treated with drugs that increase noradrenaline levels in synapses. It is therefore important that levels of noradrenaline are established before antidepressant drugs are prescribed (see pages 99–101).

Serotonin, the optimism neurotransmitter

Most people, especially if they have had any contact with mental illness or suffered any degree of depression, will have heard of serotonin. This is the neurotransmitter that the latest generation of antidepressants, called selective serotonin reuptake inhibitors (SSRIs), increases at neural synapses. Serotonin improves mood, increases serenity and optimism, and improves sleep and appetite, so low levels of this neurotransmitter can lead to severe depression.

Only 1 or 2 per cent of the body's serotonin is found in the brain. The rest is in blood platelets, mast cells which are important in the immune system and the intestine. This serotonin is kept out of the brain by the blood–brain barrier; otherwise our moods would fluctuate even more than they do.

Melatonin, which affects sleep patterns, is synthesised from serotonin in the pineal gland. This gland is known as the 'third eye' because its activity is influenced by light detected by the retina. The production of melatonin is stimulated by darkness and inhibited by light.

Endorphins

Endorphins are the most potent neurotransmitters of all and tiny amounts can have a profound effect. Endorphins are made in the brain and act not only as neurotransmitters but also as neurohormones, chemical messengers affecting nerve function in more distant parts of the brain.

The highest concentration of receptors for endorphins in the brain is in the sensory regions of the cerebrum and particular regions of the limbic system, especially the hypothalamus. Importantly, endorphins inhibit firing of neurons in the amygdala, the brain's fear and anxiety centre. Natural endorphins are released as a result of taking exercise and, unlike recreational opiate drugs, stimulate the emotional brain to find more pleasure in sex as well as friendship, food and other day-to-day activities. (The role of physical activity in overcoming mental illness is discussed on pages 189–90.)

WHAT GOES WRONG WHEN WE ARE ANXIOUS AND DEPRESSED

The autonomic nervous system

As previously pointed out, many experts working in the field of mental illness now believe that anxiety and depression reflect problems with the autonomic nervous system, the part of the nervous system that regulates the involuntary actions of the body beyond our conscious control, such as heartbeat and breathing. The autonomic nervous system comprises the nuclei in the brain stem, where neurotransmitters are secreted, and the hypothalamus which is linked to the body's master gland, the pituitary, which controls the release of hormones (see diagram page 44).

The autonomic nervous system consists of the sympathetic and parasympathetic divisions, which try to maintain our equilibrium in response to stimulating and tranquillising forces, respectively. When the sympathetic nervous system dominates, the body is said to be ready for 'fight or flight', and when the parasympathetic nervous system dominates the body is said to be in a state of 'rest and digest'.

Fight or flight vs rest and digest

The sympathetic nervous system is concerned with mobilising the body's resources to handle threats. It evolved in primates and humans from earlier mammals and is designed to cope with immediate threats, such as the appearance of a predator or other such frightening event.

When the sympathetic nervous system switches into action our primitive reptilian brain, which is concerned with our survival, takes control. We don't have time to think logically and the cerebrum is temporarily switched off. Unfortunately, this system of self-defence, which meant we were well equipped to run away from hungry bears or fight attackers in our stone-age past, can cause serious problems with our mental health in the quite different conditions of the twenty-first century.

Faced with a sudden threat, the body is mobilised in seconds by the sympathetic nervous system, as hormones bring about major physiological changes in the brain and body. The hypothalamus, pituitary and adrenal glands (often referred to as the HPA axis) are central to this response. The amygdala – the brain's fear centre – sends a signal that is carried down through the 'chain of command' from the hypothalamus and pituitary to the adrenal glands, releasing the fast-acting stress hormones adrenaline and noradrenaline and the longer-lived stress hormone cortisol, which can act for hours after release. These hormones are highly fat-soluble and readily cross the blood–brain barrier into the brain.

These hormones speed up the whole metabolic rate and have the following effects:

- The heart beats faster and stronger.

- Blood is diverted to the muscles so they become ready for action.

- The levels of glucose in the blood are increased as a source of energy.

- The bronchi (air passages) of the lungs dilate so that more oxygen can be taken in and more carbon dioxide breathed out as we burn more fuel.

- Digestion slows down as energy is diverted to more immediate needs.

- Levels of fatty acids in the blood are increased, for reasons that are not yet fully understood.

In early humans, the body would have used these heightened

physical capabilities to fight or flee, or until the parasympathetic nervous system took over, returning the body to a calm state by slowing down heart rate and breathing, relaxing the muscles and stimulating the digestion. Unfortunately, many of us experience the first part of this sequence regularly – but not the second. Part of the reason for this is that many events in the modern world, although not life-threatening, can trigger the fight-or-flight reaction: for example, an impending deadline at work, noisy neighbours or even an inflammatory remark.

Moreover, these stressful events usually don't require any physical effort to resolve. Whereas stone-age man effectively used up his stress hormones in fighting or fleeing, this is often not appropriate for us. Also, the sympathetic nervous system often dominates over the parasympathetic system for evolutionary reasons, so that we remain watchful for a time after a threatening event. Hence, not only does our sympathetic nervous system switch on inappropriately but it also often stays switched on for too long, especially if we are unable to resolve the stressful situation quickly. (If you are interested in the autonomic nervous system you'll find a helpful diagram in the 'facts' section at www.stress-anxiety-depression-support.com)

It is important to note that the stress response is a function not only of the intensity of the external 'threat' but also of the person's perception of and reaction to the threat. So why do some people react more to events than others and how is the fight-or-flight reaction linked to anxiety and depression?

Malign memories

Part of the reason why some of us react to stressful events more than others lies in the way in which the brain stores strong negative emotions such as fear, anger or disgust in the unconscious mind. The fast heartbeat and rapid breathing, the upset digestion and all the unpleasant sensations associated with, for example, a sudden threat are registered by our conscious minds, but more importantly they are registered and stored in our unconscious memory.[10] This is known as the implicit memory, centred on the amygdala (remember, this is the brain's fear centre). Such negative memory formation in the unconscious mind is thought to be facilitated by noradrenaline.[11]

At the same time, the hippocampus, which is central to the formation of conscious long-term explicit memory, fails to function properly and the short-term working memory in the prefrontal cortex is also impaired by the high levels of circulating stress hormones. This means that our intellectual or cognitive response is effectively switched off and we record the event only in the instinctive rapid-response part of the brain.

This system for storing memories in our unconscious mind – memories that can be rapidly retrieved – is thought to have evolved in our ancestors. It helped protect them from sudden threats by reminding them to avoid such situations or to help them cope better next time. It is now thought that it is powerful negative memories such as these, stored in the amygdala, which can cause an over-reaction to stress in modern humans. For example, if as a child you witnessed a violent argument between your parents and some neighbours, which you perceived to be threatening, the memory of that event may, at a subconscious level, be dictating your response to disputes with neighbours in adult life. And, of course, every time you experience such a response the powerful negative memories are amplified.

One of the most frustrating things for people who suffer from anxiety is that their emotional state often bears little relation to reality. This is because malign memories cause us to overreact badly to similar stressful events long after the original threatening event occurred. Implicit memory can generate emotions that affect our moods and interact with our thoughts so that they become illogical and irrational without us ever knowing why. In this way, malign memories, especially if they are laid down in early childhood, expose us to high levels of stress and can lead to anxiety and depression.

In some people, activation of the amygdala can occur in the absence of any real threat. High levels of cortisol, even as a result of being hungry or thirsty or physically ill, can switch on the amygdala, especially in vulnerable people. The amygdala can, in turn, switch on the HPA axis and a negative feedback loop can be established whereby the amygdala keeps sending and receiving fear signals, in turn triggering the HPA axis, which in turn triggers the amygdala. This cycle, if it happens repeatedly in the absence of stress or if the reaction is too intense or prolonged, is inappropriate and can cause panic attacks and lead to chronic anxiety states.

Many of the talking therapies used to treat anxiety and depression are aimed at accessing and redeveloping the implicit memory stored in the amygdala and teaching us how to deal with problems caused by our malign memories (see pages 132–41).

The effects of chronic stress

The changes that take place in the autonomic nervous system as a result of stress were first described by the endocrinologist Hans Selye, who based his theory on animal experiments.[12] He showed that animals exposed to unpleasant or harmful stimuli such as extreme cold go through a similar series of reactions. Recent observations on more than 30,000 human patients on whom metabolic, physiological and neuropharmacological tests have been performed suggest that similar reactions can be identified in humans.[13]

According to Selye, there are three stages to the stress response. The first stage is the 'alarm' or fight-or-flight response outlined above. Stage two is reached when stress is ongoing and the body is exposed to excessive levels of stress hormones. If this continues the body becomes progressively depleted and eventually reaches physical and mental exhaustion – stage three. Interestingly, anxiety is thought to represent the instinct to escape witnessed in Selye's experiments on animals subjected to stress, while depression is thought to reflect withdrawal, which can lead to breakdown, also known as uncoping stress (see page 65).

The negative effects of excess stress hormones

If the body frequently switches into fight-or-flight mode, or maintains a state of alert for some time, an excessive amount of stress hormones is generated. This is problematic for a number of reasons. In order to get the body back to a state of rest and digest, the parasympathetic system uses the neurotransmitters GABA and serotonin to break down or neutralise stress hormones such as noradrenaline, adrenaline and cortisol. This process depletes the brain's supply of GABA and serotonin, which are important for tranquillity and optimism respectively.

In addition, the high levels of stress hormones in themselves cause problems. The body's ongoing demand for noradrenaline can lead to levels becoming depleted, reducing our attentiveness and enthusiasm and leaving us physically and emotionally drained. Raised adrenaline levels can have longer-term effects such as high blood pressure and a greater risk of heart attack or stroke. However, it is the high levels of cortisol that most affect our cognitive function – and thus our ability to cope with life generally.

Cortisol is a necessary part of the stress response and is a key hormone in many other ways, for example it helps release energy from storage, helps maintain the correct water balance in the body, stimulates the release of endorphins and counters inflammation and allergies. However, ongoing high cortisol levels have a negative effect on the body, such as:

- Interfering with the sleep cycle by stimulating the body when it should be asleep.

- Dampening the body's inflammatory and immune responses, sometimes leading to physical illnesses, especially if the stress persists.

- Damaging and destroying neurons in the hippocampus, the brain region involved in memory and emotion. This contains its own stem cells, however, and can regenerate when stress levels fall.[14]

- Interfering with the action of some of the main neurotransmitters – serotonin, noradrenaline and dopamine.

In situations of chronic stress, cortisol continues to stimulate the locus coeruleus in the reptilian brain, increasing levels of noradrenaline. These, in turn, stimulate the brain's fear centre, the amygdala. Serotonin levels fall but, initially, noradrenaline levels in the brain remain high relative to serotonin, producing many of the symptoms of major depression. This, like most types of depression, reflects the dominance of the sympathetic nervous system over the parasympathetic system. It is important to note, however, that this situation does not apply to all types of depression. Dysthymic depression (see page 35) reflects the dominance of the parasympathetic nervous system, in which levels of serotonin are too high relative to noradrenaline.[15]

Uncoping stress and breakdown

At its most serious, chronic stress can eventually exhaust the body's noradrenaline supply and the activity of the sympathetic nervous system is maintained only by high levels of stress hormones such as adrenaline and cortisol. The excess stress hormones can, in turn, damage the brain by impeding its function directly or by increasing its susceptibility to other damaging agents, affecting our ability to think logically and hence to cope. In situations of intense or prolonged stress, the explicit memory in the hippocampus and the working short-term memory in the prefrontal cortex are also impaired.

This condition is the same as that produced in experimental animals subjected to inescapable stress observed by Hans Selye. Such animals are said to show behavioural despair. For example, if an experimental rat receives an electric shock whatever it does and can find no way of avoiding this, it will sooner or later show behavioural despair – a condition similar to what is referred to as uncoping stress in humans, a serious type of depression that is the result of chronic stress that is perceived to be inescapable. Physical illnesses such as cardiovascular, gastro-intestinal, metabolic, endocrine and immunological disorders can result from uncoping stress.[15]

In the rest of the book we help you to prevent and treat stress, anxiety and depression, empowering you to take more control of your life and mental well-being.

Chapter Four

Risk Factors – Why it's All about Strawberries and Lemons

A COMPREHENSIVE UNDERSTANDING OF ANXIETY and depression that can be used to develop effective, quick-acting medical treatments or 'magic bullets', is probably still several years away. However, it is possible to identify the main risk factors associated with our lifestyle or environment that can cause the sympathetic nervous system to switch on inappropriately or to stay switched on, leading to excess stress, anxiety and depression. We hope that an understanding of these risk factors will enable you to eliminate many of them and greatly reduce the impact of others.

Obviously, it isn't possible to change our genes, early childhood or age, but we can change the way we react to them – and many other risk factors are avoidable or preventable. Depressive illness, like cancer, is a multifactorial disease and a helpful way to think of such illnesses is as 'slot-machine diseases'. Think about playing on a slot machine. If you get one strawberry with two lemons it's no big deal; even with two strawberries in a row with one lemon, nothing happens. But if you get three strawberries in a row then you've hit the jackpot. Similarly, it is when several risk factors all apply to you that you are likely to develop anxiety or depression. In the case of anxiety and depression, the last strawberry, the one that triggers illness, can be something quite minor – the last straw.

What this means is that if you have one or two risk factors implicated in anxiety and depression, say a gene and an adverse early life experience, you would probably not develop anxiety or depression, but if a third factor arises in your life you could become ill. As we shall see, there are several 'strawberries' or risk factors for anxiety and depression, many of which are preventable. These are nearly all elements that cause stress to our minds or bodies. For example, a difficult relationship can cause stress to the mind, while a slimming diet with too few calories can cause stress to the body.

Although anxiety and depression are widely recognised as multifactorial diseases, the predictive role of high levels of stress hormones in response to frightening experiences or losses such as bereavement suggest that stress for many people is the most important factor in the subsequent onset of illness (though the illness may not start until long after the stressful event).[1] As we learnt in the previous chapter, stressful situations are likely to switch on the amygdala, with its fears and malign memories, and the sympathetic nervous system.

Studies have shown that high levels of cortisol are found in 40 to 60 per cent of depressed patients.[2] The relationship is not simple, however, in that it is not possible to say that the higher the levels of cortisol the more likely it is that there will be a depressive episode (see pages 63–4). Nevertheless, the effects of intense acute stress or chronic stress are considered to be some of the most important factors in precipitating the onset of anxiety or depression, so let us look at some of the sources of stress in our lives as we consider the different risk factors.

RISK FACTORS THAT CANNOT BE CHANGED

Making us vulnerable

Most of us are aware that people differ greatly in their ability to withstand stress. Some people can be seriously upset by apparently quite small things and are often described as being sensitive or delicate. In the most vulnerable individuals, incidents that to other people seem quite minor can lead to episodes of mental illness. Jane remembers vividly how on one occasion her father, who enjoyed shooting bottles from a wall with a rifle, became seriously depressed for weeks after he accidentally killed a sparrow that flew across the path of the shot. On the other hand some people can cope with very distressing situations and emerge relatively unscathed. So why are some of us so much more vulnerable than others? Are we simply preprogrammed by our genes so that some of us are simply born that way, or are other factors in our early life experiences involved?

In our genes?

Many of us who suffer from anxiety and depression worry that it is in our genes, hence we are going to suffer for the rest of our lives and possibly pass on our predisposition to our children. There is indeed increasing evidence of the role of genes in anxiety and depression, but it is worth remembering that this is just one of the risk factors and there are lots of others that we can avoid so that we don't 'hit the jackpot' and become ill. Both humans and experimental laboratory rats show marked individual differences in the way they respond to stress, reflecting differences in genetic make-up. Studies comparing identical twins (who are genetically identical) and non-identical twins (who are not) show that about 50 per cent of the variation in cortisol levels between people is determined by their genes, which means that the remaining 50 per cent is determined by other factors, some of which you can control.[3]

It has been suggested that certain genes may be involved in the production and regulation of serotonin and cortisol, though the particular genes responsible have not been identified. In the long term, it is hoped that understanding the genetic components of psychiatric disorders will lead to the development of new treatments. In the short term, whatever genetic make-up you have inherited, it is important to realise that good genes can be turned on and bad genes turned off (see below). For example, this may be brought about simply by changing what we choose to eat (see Chapter 10). Moreover, as discussed in Chapter 3, genes can actually help the brain to relearn and rewire itself. In relation to the brain and mind, it has been stated by Nobel prizewinning neuroscientist Eric Kandel that genes are not simply the determinants of behaviour: they are also servants of the environment.[4]

Switching genes on and off

Recent information suggests that our genetic predisposition to illnesses such as anxiety and depression is also related to information stored in proteins and other chemicals that surround and adhere to DNA (epigenetics). Like DNA, these chemicals are inherited.[5] One of the effects of these chemicals is to 'switch' genes on or off, which is why some people with a predisposition to an illness succumb to that illness while others do not. In the case of bipolar disorder, for example, it has been suggested that epigenetic differences between identical twins may account for the 30–70 per cent of cases where only one twin has the illness.[6] Factors such as diet have been shown to be crucially important in epigenetics: two experimental animals bred to have identical genes develop quite differently if their mother is given different diets during pregnancy. The early embryo is particularly susceptible to having genes switched on or switched off by epigenetic influences. Researchers also believe that characteristics developed as a result of factors such as the mother's diet during pregnancy can be passed on to the offspring, so epigenetics can be responsible for quite dramatic changes from one generation to the next, whereas genetic changes, in contrast, occur over many generations. We shall deal with lifestyle and food factors that may affect gene expression in Chapters 9 and 10.

What this means is that even if you have inherited genes that predispose you to anxiety and depression, by improving your diet and eliminating lifestyle factors that generate stress you can greatly reduce the influence of bad genes and even switch them off, while switching on your protective genes.

Sex

There are significant differences between men and women in their response to stress and their vulnerability to mood disorders.[7] Women tend naturally to have higher levels of stress hormones than men and they are also more vulnerable to anxiety, depression and even

Alzheimer's disease. It is thought to be the male hormone testosterone that protects against stress,[8] and there is some evidence that the sex differences in vulnerability to depressive illness become more marked at puberty.[9] High oestrogen and progesterone levels during pregnancy, however, are thought to give some temporary protection to women.[10] Recent evidence from PET scans shows that men's brains produce serotonin at a faster rate than those of women.[11]

Age

Anxiety and depression can begin at any age. There is concern about the number of young children who are affected now. Many conditions first appear in the late teens to early twenties. Some people who are affected may continue to be affected, on and off, for the rest of their lives. Others never suffer again. Depression and anxiety can affect menopausal women, andropausal men and some elderly people, but this is thought to reflect changing life circumstances rather than a fundamental biological process. It is worth remembering from the human function curve discussed in Chapter 2 that we all need some degree of stimulation (eustress) in our lives and that boredom and loneliness can cause just as many problems as too much pressure. We discuss this further in Chapter 9 on lifestyle changes.

Influences on the unborn baby

In the past, great efforts were made to protect pregnant women from stress. Even in the 1950s they were encouraged to rest a lot and were protected from bad news and stressful situations. Amazingly, science is now showing that there were sound reasons for this. There is now strong evidence that adverse physical or social events that generate intense or chronic stress in pregnant animals or humans can affect the response of the unborn baby to stress and predispose it to excessive or inappropriate anxiety and depressive illness later in life.[12]

Some baby monkeys are born abnormally fearful and anxious, and this happens with human babies too. Such babies react strongly to any stress, including changes to their usual routine, and they find difficulty throughout their lives in situations that others find unchallenging. The extent to which this vulnerability is genetic or is related to the effects of stress experienced by the mother on her unborn baby is not known. It has been suggested that when a mother's stress is transmitted to her unborn baby, a pattern is established that can last throughout life, with the sympathetic nervous system switching on too readily.[13]

There is also evidence that the increased anxiety and exaggerated stress responses of such affected individuals can lead not only to depressive illnesses in later life but also to physical disorders such as hypertension (high blood pressure) and insulin resistance (vulnerability to type 2 diabetes). These conditions can, in turn, affect brain function. Clearly there is nothing we can do about what happened to our mothers before we were born, but we can minimise the stress of pregnant women today, to prevent this effect being passed on to future generations.

Newborn babies and breast-feeding

There is now considerable evidence that newborn babies are capable of significant perception and can interact with their environment from the earliest days of life.[14] The long, complex process of socialisation begins at this time, as the prefrontal cortex of the brain develops.

A woman's response to stress is suppressed during breast-feeding, and all the evidence is that breast-feeding is protective of the mental health of both mother and child. Indeed, some evidence suggests that breast-feeding, combined with a diet high in nutrients such as omega-3 and -6 fatty acids, vitamins and minerals, protects against post-natal depression.[15]

Family members who wish to help should remember that their principal role is to support the mother to nurture her baby rather than making the new baby their priority. Breast-feeding helps to reinforce these family relationships.

Early life experiences

There is much evidence that early life experiences are important in making us vulnerable to anxiety and depression.[16]

Separation

Interpersonal relationships between mother and child appear to be particularly important. Baby rats that are separated from their mother for long periods of time and are deprived of close contact and interaction with her have a higher response to stress in later life.[17] The length of the separation appears to be crucial. It now seems that in humans too there is a critical neonatal period in which disruption of maternal care, whereby mother and baby are separated for long periods of time (not just on a daily basis), can predispose the young to overreact to stress and hence to suffer from anxiety and depression later in life.

If young animals have serious infections which increase the levels of circulating stress hormones such as cortisol, similar problems can arise. Again, it is thought that such situations give rise to stress and that this can affect the sensitivity of the sympathetic nervous system throughout life – which can in turn affect metabolism and cardiovascular function in adults.

John Bowlby trained as a child psychiatrist and psychoanalyst in the 1930s and 1940s and in 1969 to 1980 published his seminal work on attachment (called 'attachment theory') between mother and child, and how the loss of this relationship was an important factor in sadness and depression.[18] His findings were based on direct observations of children and experimental animals. He identified the powerful influence of the parent–child relationship that is established early in development and goes on to influence all further interactions. He observed that a six-month-old monkey's reaction to separation from its mother is similar to that of a child. There is initially agitation, with screams and crying and a loss of interest in people or toys. The infant subsequently becomes unresponsive and lethargic, and this depressed state persists and is made worse by unfamiliar surroundings. Monkeys that are separated from their mothers at birth and are reared in small groups of other baby monkeys develop strong attachments to each other, but still tend to be more anxious, less secure and more vulnerable to anxiety and depression in later life. Recent work confirms this.[19]

The biological basis of attachment theory appears to be linked to the development of the prefrontal cortex, which, as we learnt in Chapter 3, is the part of the brain that enables us to empathise and to restrain primitive emotional impulses and deal with stress.

Allan Schore, the famous neuropsychoanalyst and a pioneer in integrating social, biological, psychological and psychoanalytical theory, uses Bowlby's ideas as an overarching model. Indeed, he has been called the American Bowlby. In his famous book, *Affect Regulation and the Origin of the Self*, he argues that the development of the prefrontal cortex of the brain depends on a positive emotional experience between the child and parent figure.[20] This causes endorphins and dopamine to be released which, in turn, cause parts of the brain, especially the prefrontal cortex, to grow as well as facilitating connections to develop with other parts of the brain. The prefrontal cortex does not develop automatically, and studies have shown that neglected babies such as Romanian orphans have smaller prefrontal cortexes than normal.[21] In other words the looks and smiles of a loving parent are the most vital stimulus to the growth of the social, emotionally intelligent human brain.

Although we cannot change our own early life experiences, we can learn to break patterns of behaviour that result from them and that may be generating stress and predisposing us to anxiety and depression (see pages 139–41).

Fostering emotional security

We should all try to prevent children being affected by adverse early life experiences. This does not mean that parents have to give up work or that they should be overprotective, but they should spend as much quality time as they can with their children, showing them love and affection and giving them as much emotional security as possible.

Unfortunately, patterns of depression can be repeated through the generations. Parents with a secure childhood generally bring up secure children, while depressed or anxious parents tend to have offspring who also suffer from these conditions.[22] Post-natal depression can be particularly important in maintaining intergenerational anxiety and depression, especially if the mother neglects or rejects her child while she is ill and there is no other person to nurture it.

Parental control and pressure

Many studies show that depressive illnesses can result from having controlling, demanding parents as a child.[23] An example is a family in which any achievement is met with some degree of criticism: for instance, a child who tells their parents how high their marks were in an examination, only to be asked if they came top and if not, why not? Such a child is left with the impression that they must do better next time. High marks and outstanding performance are required before the child receives love or attention. Depressives are also more likely as children to have been subjected to negative words, like bad, stupid, inadequate, useless and, worst of all, unwanted. It is thought that in Britain at least one child in ten is exposed to such hypercriticism.[24]

Managing change and competition in the family

Changes from familiar to unfamiliar social circumstances in children younger than five can cause considerable stress, especially in vulnerable children, and there can also be a long-term adverse effect on memory.

Remember that children like to have a routine, so always try to introduce change gradually. If you have children already and are expecting another baby, prepare and involve the older child in this so that they don't feel rejected because most of your attention is now on the new baby.

Children equate attention with love. It is important to treat all children as fairly and equally as possible. Although some people have favourites, it is simply not fair to let the children know this. It is far better to engender love, not rivalry, between siblings. Some parents cause terrible harm that can go on through the generations because they try to divide and rule their family to give themselves a central, powerful position.

Sudden threats

In addition to chronic stress caused by a lack of appropriate nurturing, there is much evidence that malign memories laid down in childhood as a result of bad experiences during infancy and early childhood, exposing the brain to increased levels of stress hormones, can have long-lasting consequences.[25]

Setting boundaries

All children need to know where the boundaries are and to be given firm, consistent guidelines on what is acceptable and unacceptable behaviour, but hitting children or physically abusing them is counter-productive, as is screaming and yelling at them. The high levels of stress generated switch off their human brains and make them behave like naughty little animals!

We should all remember that any incidents that cause young children to experience strong emotions such as intense fear, anger or disgust are likely to be locked in their memories, with the potential to cause them mental health problems later in life.

Several men and women we know are aware that they overreact badly in situations where they are disciplined or even mildly told off, especially by women. Clearly this can be particularly difficult in modern work settings. In each case their mothers suffered badly from premenstrual tension and as children they were likely to be shouted at apparently unpredictably.

Similarly, the children of alcoholic fathers who witnessed violent or abusive behaviour to their mothers can overreact to even a hint of aggression.

CASE HISTORY: Richard

Richard became ill every time he went to London because that was where he had lived with a violent alcoholic father. Within months of moving back to the city to live he was suffering from all sorts of heart problems because his sympathetic nervous system was switched on almost permanently, triggered by memories in his unconscious mind. Once he had therapy and understood what was causing the problem and was helped to deal with the past and its effects on him, his health improved dramatically. He now lives in London.

Clearly the physical or sexual abuse of children, which is likely to cause intense fear and in many cases disgust, will have the potential to affect their mental health adversely throughout their lives. Other events in childhood can also affect people throughout their lives. For example, if you were bitten by a dog as a child, you may have implanted in your unconscious that all dogs will bite and believe this implicitly, though logic tells you that most dogs are friendly. It can be extremely hard to break the habitual reaction, even though you are conscious that your response is inappropriate to the situation. Many anxiety states such as agoraphobia (a fear of open spaces) or claustrophobia (a fear of being in a confined space) are thought to be caused in this way.

All early adverse life events are thought to have the potential for long-lasting detrimental effects on brain function, which in some cases can persist for life. This is probably related to the increased sensitivity caused to the HPA axis and the ease with which it switches on the sympathetic nervous system (see pages 59–61). The precise processes involved in such early programming are still not fully understood, though sites on the hypothalamus are thought to be involved, as well as the prefrontal cortex. If you are still affected by such childhood experiences you are likely to find some type of talking therapy helpful (see Chapter 7).

Protecting your children

If you suffer badly from premenstrual tension or post-natal depression try at all costs not to take it out on the children. Seek help and ensure that your partner knows and can take over in situations in which you feel you might lose control, or find a relative or friend to help until you feel better able to cope. If you have a problem with drugs or alcohol seek help and do everything possible not to let your problems affect your children.

It is clear, then, that some people will be more vulnerable to anxiety and depression than others because of a combination of genetics, epigenetics, sex, age and early life experiences, over which we have limited or no control. This raises the question: what risk factors can we influence?

RISK FACTORS THAT CAN BE ELIMINATED OR REDUCED

Psychosocial factors

Losses and change

We all experience losses throughout our lives. For example, we lose our childhood innocence and beliefs in such things as tooth fairies and Father Christmas, and later we experience the loss of familiar surroundings and many friends when we leave school or college. Some people suffer much more damaging losses, such as family breakdown or the death of a loved one. These early experiences can affect our future behaviour unless we learn to adapt and cope and come to understand that loss and change does not have to be entirely negative. Some losses can lead to gains. For example, leaving one job is often followed by an even better position, and leaving one group of friends often leads to making many new ones.

Nevertheless, losses, especially the severe and permanent breakdown of a confiding relationship through bereavement or divorce, or a loss of status as in employment situations, can be important factors in triggering depressive illness, sometimes weeks or months later. Coming to terms with such events always takes time, but it can be helped by counselling. It is always worth seeking such help if you know you are vulnerable to depression or anxiety, particularly if there is an experience of serious loss earlier in life (see Chapter 7).

Giving birth and post-natal depression

Ten to 15 per cent of all women develop some form of post-natal depression lasting more than two weeks after giving birth. Without the right treatment this can last for months or sometimes longer.[26] While many new mothers experience 'baby blues' at some time during the two weeks after giving birth, when mood swings are common, this usually passes in a day or two. This is not the same as post-natal depression, which is an illness associated with severe mood disorder.

As with depression generally, there are many interrelated physical, psychological and social factors that contribute to post-natal depression. These include a history of depression, a family history of mental disorders, a lack of practical and emotional support, partner relationship difficulties, stressful life events such as the death of a loved one or moving house, an unplanned pregnancy, a prolonged or difficult labour, problems with the baby's health, and a lack of sleep. Poor or inadequate nutrition is also increasingly recognised as a factor, as discussed further in Chapter 10. Not everyone has the same symptoms; each person's experience is unique. Post-natal depression is treatable, given the right medical help, support and time, as we saw at the end of Janet's story.

Post-natal depression can be particularly important as a factor in maintaining intergenerational problems of anxiety and depression, especially if the mother cannot relate to her baby or they are separated in the first weeks or months of life.[27] Breast-feeding can be protective, but the mother must be well nourished (see Chapter 10).

Social environment

Humans are naturally social animals, but the social environment can be a potent source of stress. Monkeys at the bottom of the social hierarchy have higher cortisol levels (with flattened daily cycles) than more dominant animals.[28] This is thought to reflect stress and anxiety related to the need to obtain a share of scarce resources, as well as a general lack of control over their situation.

In humans, children from lower socio-economic groups have higher cortisol levels than those from higher groups.[29] Stress is also higher in men from lower socio-economic groups.[30] Unsurprisingly, health generally is poorer in lower socio-economic groups.[31] High emotionality, shyness and low self-esteem (the value we place on ourselves) are thought to be key factors in this.

Social adversity and physical threats

Chronic social adversity, such as living in crime-ridden run-down estates, can cause increased stress levels, which has been linked to high rates of depressive illness. Threats of physical harm, whether real or perceived, can generate considerable stress, leading to intense anxiety and depression, especially in vulnerable people. We discuss the things you can do to help minimise this factor in Chapter 9 and what society needs to do in Chapter 11.

An appropriate education

There is a lot that can be done to help children, in addition to parental and family support. We need an education system designed to equip children to lead happy, productive lives, recognising that we need lots of people who are good at doing things (and relatively few academics capable of thinking great thoughts). Many children with natural enthusiasms become disaffected as our system tries to force them all into a similar academic straightjacket.

If we are to improve children's self-esteem, we need to encourage them to develop whatever abilities and interests they have, whether that is sport, dancing, design technology, cooking, art or mathematics. Unfortunately, in the UK the snobbery, including that of government, that seems to think the only measure of educational success is a university place is unhelpful. On the other hand the inverted snobbery of some teachers in some state schools that says it is OK to recognise particular aptitudes in sport or music by putting them in the first team or the school orchestra, but not streaming children to study mathematics or science, can cause some academic children to become bored and depressed.

Self-esteem

People with low self-esteem generally have been found to have higher levels of the stress hormone cortisol and smaller hippocampuses (explicit memory) and to be much more prone to depressive illnesses than those with higher self-esteem.[32] A lack of self-esteem is highly correlated with depressive symptoms and has been shown to affect health generally, as well as life satisfaction and life expectancy.

There is much we can do as individuals to improve our self-esteem (see Chapter 9) and we discuss what society can do to help in Chapter 11.

Achievement

Many people with depressive illness are unduly self-critical and are afflicted by feelings of unworthiness, inferiority, failure and guilt. They are often, in fact, high achievers who are hard on themselves and plagued by a fear of disapproval, criticism and lack of acceptance by others. They may set themselves impossibly high standards and strive for achievement and perfection, so they are often highly competitive and hard working, making huge demands on themselves yet never finding lasting satisfaction even if they succeed. Employers who write off someone with a depressive illness as being unable to make a useful contribution have often failed to understand the nature of the condition in such individuals. There is much we can do as adults to deal with such problems, as discussed in Chapter 9.

> ### A happy child is a brighter child
>
> We should all try to remember that children who are happy and
> secure are likely to have much better memory function and
> cognitive ability than children who are unhappy and insecure.
> Support and positive interest are far more likely to help children
> do well at school than threats and pressure.

Materialism

The adoption of materialistic values can make people, especially high
achievers, vulnerable to depressive illness. Studies in fifteen countries
have shown that people who place a high value on money, possessions, appearances (social or physical) and fame are more at risk of depression, anxiety, substance abuse and personality disorders.[33] All
humans need to feel secure, competent and part of a community. Ma-
terialists are less likely to recognise this. They have been shown to have
low self-esteem, to feel they lack control over their lives, to feel insecure and to lack intimate relationships. In the words of Oliver James:
'Trapped on a treadmill of prize-chasing, from early childhood they
have only ever looked outwards for definition. Sooner or later, however much money they have earned or however powerful they have
become, their inner sense of worthlessness and impotence catches up
with them.'[33] There is much more about this in Chapter 9.

Physiological factors

In Chapters 7 and 9 there is much advice on how to help yourself or
others to develop coping strategies to prevent, treat and overcome
depressive illness, based on the psychosocial factors discussed above.
Depressive illnesses can be purely biological, however, and related to
the side effects of medication taken for other conditions, for example,
or to the introduction of an additive in a favourite food. So let us look
briefly at some of the physical and chemical factors that can lead to
anxiety and depression.

The physical environment

It is important to recognise that our bodies can produce the same stress hormones in response to physical stress as they do in response to psychosocial factors, especially in conditions likely to threaten the regulation of our internal metabolism (homeostasis). This is important because people often ignore the basic physiological signals that can build up their stress levels and adversely affect their mental well-being.

Adequate food and water intake

A lack of food and water can cause stress levels to rise significantly. Many people fail to drink enough water. If we become dehydrated there will be a specific response that makes us feel thirsty and, importantly, this is accompanied by a rise in stress hormones such as cortisol.

In the West, the main risk is probably to people on slimming diets, especially if they are extreme with restricted calorie intakes. Diets too high in protein, especially animal protein, such as the Atkins Diet, are of particular concern and some diets are now thought to be deficient in essential fatty acids and essential minerals such as iodine, lithium, magnesium and zinc. The relationship between diet and depression is considered more fully in Chapter 10.

Food additives

Some additives can affect the brain, especially in situations where the blood–brain barrier is not fully effective, and there is strong evidence of its increased 'leakiness' in individuals affected by stress,[34] by chemicals such as organophosphates,[35] or as a result of alcohol abuse.[36]

To take one example, glutamate (the main excitory neurotransmitter – see page 55) is normally manufactured in the body from protein, but we can take in excessively large amounts by consuming food containing monosodium glutamate, which is usually known by its initials MSG and is sometimes marketed as 'extra meaty flavour'. Some parts of the brain are particularly vulnerable to glutamate damage caused by excessive excitory activity and it has been suggested that both aspartic acid (or aspartate) and glutamic acid (or glutamate) – the 'acidic amino acids' which are added to many fast foods and drinks – are capable of destroying neurons when present in excessive amounts in the brain.[37] Aspartame is the main man-made sugar replacement that is used in 'diet' or 'low-calorie' drinks and other products such as chewing gum. We consider the importance of dietary additives and substances further in Chapter 10.

Caffeine

Similarly, increased alertness or anxiety can be caused by the effect of caffeine in blocking receptors that normally inhibit glutamate release. Caffeine also inhibits the effect of GABA (the main inhibitory neurotransmitter – see page 56) on GABA receptors, which is one of the processes that explains its stimulatory properties. It is worth considering that many of us use caffeine drinks such as tea, coffee or colas as our main source of hydration on a daily basis.

Temperature

Excessive heat or cold causes considerable stress and is associated with high levels of circulating cortisol. Simple ways of avoiding such problems are discussed further in Chapter 9.

Noise and light pollution

These are factors well known to increase stress. Noise has been used to intimidate enemies since the battle of Jericho as described in the Old Testament of the Bible, and it is still used as an instrument of intimidation and torture.

We have evolved to respond rapidly to sudden loud noises such as the roar of a wild animal, and loud noises trigger a clear 'startle' response in babies. Our response to noise allows us to go from deep sleep to be ready for fight or flight in a matter of seconds, triggering the production of stress hormones. The high level of noise in modern society can be a particularly important factor contributing to chronic stress. Distress can be caused by noisy neighbours, traffic and aircraft noise.

Also, in modern urban environments light pollution from street lighting or advertisements can cause considerable stress. It can make it difficult to sleep, because the pineal gland fails to produce enough melatonin when there is not total darkness (see page 58).

Lack of natural daylight

Most of us, not just sufferers of SAD (see page 37) feel much better mentally and emotionally during long sunny days. We discuss some of the things that can help in Chapter 9.

Time patterns

Our levels of stress hormones, such as cortisol, normally vary throughout the day by a factor of up to eight times. The cycle is synchronised to solar time by our eyes. The pattern generally reflects our daily cycle of rest and activity, so levels in humans generally peak in the early morning and fall gradually after midday. This explains why some people suffering from depressive illness feel so much worse in the morning and somewhat better in the evening. About 50 per cent of people with depression have flattened daily patterns of cortisol, however, with high levels in the evening. Chronic stress can result not only in elevated stress hormones but also in a loss of the daily rhythm, both of which can further disturb brain function. There can be severe disruption of the daily rhythm in major or endogenous depression (and Alzheimer's disease).

Travel across time zones or changes in activity and sleep patterns (working night shifts, for example) require rephasing of the HPA axis (see page 60) and this is generally a slow process – often taking up to a week. Disturbing sleep patterns generally can be detrimental. Many studies show the importance of sleep as a restorative (see page 190).

We discuss what you can do to avoid this type of stress in Chapter 9.

Pollution

Several heavy metals and thousands of man-made chemicals have been shown to affect brain function by blocking receptors for neurotransmitters such as noradrenaline. We discuss this further, including simple ways of avoiding exposure to harmful substances, in Chapter 9.

Physical illness and infection

Most physical illnesses, especially if they are associated with pain or discomfort, can cause a great deal of stress which can in turn precipitate depression.

Many infectious illnesses, including those caused by viruses such as the Epstein-Barr virus, which is responsible for glandular fever, can cause depression. Viruses can disrupt the production of essential fatty acids, which are necessary for brain function, especially eicosapentaenoic acid or EPA (see pages 222–41). Some viruses have evolved methods of preventing EPA production because EPA can kill viruses directly and can also be converted into powerful antiviral substances. Without EPA, invading viruses can reproduce rapidly and cause extensive damage to cells and tissues. They effectively block the enzyme that is involved in the production of long-chained polyunsaturated fatty acids (LC-PUFAs), especially EPA, from simpler omega-3 and omega-6 fatty acids (see further in Chapter 10).

When we are ill, the body also produces toxic chemicals to fight infection. For example, tryptophan, instead of being converted to serotonin in the brain, can be changed to quinolinic acid to attack infectious agents. Quinolinic acid is a powerful neurotoxin, however, and can cause mental illness. Remember those films where the heroine was delirious until her fever broke. At that point her levels of quinolinic acid fell and she returned to normal.

In some patients, depressive illness mainly reflects chronic infections, such as HIV/AIDS or other viruses, or bacterial or fungal infections. The depressive illness may be partly a result of the production of quinolinic acid and other neurotoxins rather than imbalances of neurotransmitters. The patient may then be suffering from the combined effect of too little neurotransmitter and too much neurotoxin. In the case of AIDS, the virus lowers the levels of the enzyme glutathione peroxidase (GTP) which is crucial for our immune system.[38] In trying to restore this, the body consumes tryptophan and glutamine from which GTP is made, helping trigger depression.

Problems with the digestive tract can also result in depression, probably because of a failure to absorb essential nutrients. Coeliac disease, in which the patient is unable to tolerate gluten found in wheat, rye, barley and in some cases oats, is commonly associated with depression, which is resolved once a suitable diet is introduced. As many as one in 100 Caucasians may suffer from this condition although estimates vary. It can be diagnosed by a simple blood test, but it often remains undiagnosed and unsuspected for years. We always ask our patients, especially if they are excessively thin, to have a test for coeliac disease. We know several people in their fifties or sixties who have suffered with depression all their lives and been treated for mental illness, including with electroconvulsive therapy, who were found to have coeliac disease and who made a full recovery from their depression once they were on a sound dietary regime.

Side effects of medication

Many types of medication can cause anxiety and depression, not least those that are closely related to cortisol and are used as anti-inflammatory drugs to treat allergic and auto-immune diseases; there are too many such drugs to list here. With some medications a high proportion of patients might be affected, with others very few are affected. Some high-oestrogen contraceptives can lower serotonin levels in the brain and contribute to one type of depression, for example. Many chemotherapeutic drugs used in the treatment of cancer can also lead to depression. Some anti-malarial preparations can induce severe depression, even in people with no previous history of the condition. Jane saw one of her colleagues, an able and confident man well used to travelling the world and dealing with difficult situations, reduced to fearful anxiety and depression with thoughts of suicide after just a few days of taking a powerful anti-malarial drug. He recovered quickly once he stopped taking the drug. We discuss this further in Chapter 5 concerning obtaining an accurate diagnosis.

Recreational drugs

Many recreational drugs (both legal, such as alcohol and tobacco, and illegal, such as cocaine) work by temporarily increasing levels of 'feel good' neurotransmitters such as GABA, serotonin and especially dopamine at synapses in the brain. Unfortunately, these neurotransmitters are then excreted by the body so that levels fall to lower than normal. The 'low' after taking drugs such as cocaine, ecstasy or alcohol can cause intense depression, including thoughts of suicide. We have seen strong young men weeping and talking of suicide after just one or two episodes of taking recreational drugs. A vicious circle can easily be established whereby the drug (known as 'the hair of the dog' in the case of alcohol) is used to treat the resulting depression, reinforcing the condition. The problems are likely to intensify with prolonged use as individuals come to tolerate their drug so that they need higher and higher quantities to produce the desired effect.

The withdrawal effects of alcohol cause depression because alcohol over-stimulates the production of serotonin and GABA in the brain and these are subsequently lost in urine. Withdrawal from cocaine is associated with greatly reduced dopamine levels and particularly intense depression.

Many of the people turning to drugs and alcohol may be trying to relieve their distress by self-medicating. Unfortunately, few medical professionals seem to be aware or concerned about the underlying causes of depressive illnesses and addiction and they tend simply to treat the symptoms with further drugs. For example, alcoholics are generally treated with benzodiazepines (the drugs that led Jane to abuse alcohol) because they work at the same receptor in the brain! Moreover, many patients we have talked to who sought treatment for depressive illness were not asked by their doctor or psychiatrist if they could be suffering withdrawal symptoms from recreational drugs. They were simply treated with more (prescription) drugs which can alter or mask symptoms, as happened to Janet.

The problems that can be caused by recreational drugs can be demonstrated by considering the effects of cannabis, as outlined in the box overleaf. We have chosen this drug because links between cannabis and mental health are very topical: recent reports in the media suggest that regular use of cannabis can more than double the chances of suffering psychotic illnesses. The reports were based on data compiled from 35 different studies, and published in *The Lancet*, which shows that taking the drug just once increases the risk of mental illness by 41 per cent.[39] For frequent users, this rose to between 50 per cent and 200 per cent. Scientists found that heavy cannabis users were the most likely to suffer a psychotic breakdown marked by delusions, hallucinations or disordered thoughts.

Around 20 per cent of young adults claim to take cannabis at least once a week and around 40 per cent are believed to have tried it at some time in their lives.

Cannabis – some facts[40]

* Cannabis contains tetrahydrocannabinol (THC) which is an hallucinogen and sedative.

* A cannabis user may experience sensations of changed reality as brain circuits normally used for dreaming are stimulated, so that colours and sounds may seem more intense. The main features are impairment of consciousness, a distorted sense of the passage of time, and a dream-like euphoria, progressing to fragmented thought processes and hallucinations.[41]

* Cannabis disrupts co-ordination, balance and reaction time, and after a while users feel depressed, anxious, fearful, panicky or paranoid.

* Cannabis eventually impairs the ability to form memories, recall events, and shift attention from one thing to another.

* Cannabis users who have taken high doses of the drug may experience acute psychosis, and this can affect individuals with no history of such severe mental illness.

* A new brain-scanning technique shows that cannabis disrupts the brain in the same way as schizophrenia. According to Dr Manzar Ashtari of the Albert Einstein College of Medicine, New York, 'the type of damage in cannabis smokers' brains is exactly the same as that in schizophrenia and in exactly the same place in the brain'.[42]

STRAWBERRIES TO LEMONS

Whatever the mood disorder, whether chronic anxiety or bipolar disorder, there are now thought to be similar components – a genetic/epigenetic component, early life experiences and/or intergenerational problems – all of which are risk factors that cannot be changed, though we can use talking therapies to develop coping strategies and reduce their impact greatly.

Many other factors, whether social or physical, can be eliminated or their effects greatly reduced. They are the strawberries we can change to lemons, to help prevent and treat anxiety and depression. In Chapter 9 we discuss how we can improve our mental well-being by making changes to our lifestyle and diet and in Chapter 11 we consider what we can do as a society.

Part Two

*

TREATING ANXIETY AND DEPRESSION

If you are suffering from anxiety or depression it is important that you receive medical help and support. In this section of the book we explain what you can expect from health professionals. We discuss the various treatments that are now available and help you to find the best for your particular problem. We emphasise how important it is to obtain an accurate diagnosis. Our aim is to provide you with clear guidance on finding your way through mental health care systems to ensure you receive the best possible treatments and overcome your difficulties.

Chapter Five

··

Getting the Best Treatment

SEEING YOUR FAMILY DOCTOR

IF YOU ARE SUFFERING from anxiety or depression it is important that you are helped, and usually your family doctor or GP is the first port of call in most Western countries. In the UK, family doctors generally can refer you to counsellors, therapists and psychiatrists and they have links with social support services which you can access depending on your circumstances. So here are some suggestions to make sure you receive useful help and advice to treat your illness. The approach might cost the health service more in the short term but over the medium to longer term there is the potential to save much time and money and importantly to greatly reduce human suffering.

The right family doctor for you

Remember that family doctors are essentially professional human biologists trained to diagnose illness and to treat symptoms rather than to identify underlying causes. In addition to their general knowledge of medicine they usually have particular interests, which can range from childhood infectious illnesses to heart disease. If you are suffering from anxiety or depression it is important to find a doctor with some knowledge of and interest in mood disorders. Many practices now have several doctors, so ask if there is a doctor (or senior nurse) in the practice with a special interest in anxiety and depression. If you hear of others who have been helped by their doctors, find out more and try to register with one with a good reputation in the field. If you need to change doctor, explain your reasons, without criticism or unpleasantness, and thank your doctor for any help they have given to you or your family in the past.

Some GPs now practise integrated medicine and use both conventional and alternative and complementary therapies. The best practices now employ psychological therapists and counsellors or have access to them. In some practices there will be groups facilitated by a psychologist that you might consider joining after your individual treatment is completed. Try if possible to find such a practice.

The consultation

When you visit your doctor, remember that they have only a small amount of time, usually between five and ten minutes to see you and make a diagnosis. If you think it would be helpful, take a supporter with you. It might help if they take notes; it is difficult to remember everything that was said in a consultation. Help your doctor by being as clear as possible about your symptoms and whether or not you have experienced them in the past. If possible give other information such as the situations that trigger episodes of anxiety or depression. Have you recently suffered a painful loss or other stressful event? Are you affected at particular times of the year, for example, especially during the winter months? If you are a woman, tell them if your symptoms are particularly intense at certain times of the month or not.

Once you have described your symptoms, you may be asked to fill in a questionnaire based on the Diagnostic and Statistical Manual (see page 33). From this the doctor will try to evaluate your assessment of how you are feeling. Often such subjective tests are the only diagnostic tool used before you are prescribed medication. It is important, however, that you don't see your doctor only to be sent away with some standard pills that may or may not help. Bear in mind, as we discussed in Chapters 2 and 3, that there are many different types of anxiety and depression, involving different parts of the brain, different circuits and different neurotransmitters. The idea that all patients with a mood disorder will benefit from the same type of drug that simply boosts one neurotransmitter, serotonin for example, is clearly over-simplistic.

Chronic anxiety frequently involves overactivity of several parts of the brain, including the frontal lobes, whereas the hallmark of endogenous or major depression is too little activity in the prefrontal lobes (behind the eyes) and the parietal lobes (on the side of the brain towards the top), with too much activity in the emotional brain or limbic system. In some cases the particular circuit and neurotransmitter concerned has been identified. Many doctors now consider OCD to be a neurological rather than a mental disorder.[1] In OCD, in which obsessions and compulsions are so severe that they disrupt normal life, a dopamine circuit is thought to be involved. This circuit, which connects the black area in the brain stem to the striatum in the limbic system which controls automatic movement and an area in the frontal lobe of the brain concerned with planning, is thought to be overactive in people with OCD.

It is important, therefore, that the doctor prescribes the best drug for you and at the correct dose, but unfortunately most use no other diagnostic tests and it is unfortunately often just a 'suck it and see' process depending on your doctor's experience and biases. This approach can be a particular problem in cases of depression, where most drugs usually take two to three weeks to begin working. The wrong medication may be prescribed and if it does not appear to be working it may be changed to another type or the dose may be changed. This can lead to months – even years – of trial and error.

Sleeping tablets including benzodiazepines may be prescribed. We know of some cases where patients have ended up taking so much medication that it is difficult to distinguish the effects of medication, including withdrawal effects from sleeping tablets and tranquillisers, from the symptoms of the original illness. Remember the problems Jane had after being prescribed benzodiazepines.

DIAGNOSIS

Physical causes

Clearly one of the first things that is essential in dealing with mental illness is better diagnosis and initially all physical illnesses need to be ruled out. Your doctor should check to ensure that the symptoms of anxiety and depression are not part of some other medical condition.[2] Studies suggest that physical illness may account for more than 10 per cent of patients with symptoms of mental disorder.[3] Simple blood tests can be carried out to check for coeliac or thyroid disease, which can give rise to many of the symptoms of depression, and it is relatively cheap to check for deficiencies and imbalances in minerals such as calcium and magnesium, which can also give rise to many of the symptoms of mental illness. Some types of heart murmurs can cause anxiety, so your doctor should determine whether this is the case.

All this may involve a physical examination and some blood tests. If possible, wait for the results of these before returning to see your doctor. If a physical condition is diagnosed, take the medication prescribed and follow other advice – for example by adopting a gluten-exclusion diet in the case of coeliac disease – to see if your symptoms of anxiety and depression clear up.

Several of Janet's patients who believed that they had a mental health problem because of their violent mood swings before their periods have been diagnosed with progesterone deficiencies – but only after they had insisted on being tested. They have all made excellent recoveries although many of their lives had been seriously damaged by the time their problem was diagnosed. Although not every case of premenstrual tension or post-natal depression or psychosis will be caused by a simple deficiency in progesterone, it is worth checking for this. It is also worth checking for deficiencies or imbalances of zinc, magnesium, iron, omega-3 fatty acids and the B vitamins in cases of post-natal depression – and depression or anxiety associated with premenstrual tension.

If you have a condition that you think has a physical component but is undiagnosed it is worth persuading your doctor to consult one of the laboratories that serves Harley Street in London, such as Biolab or TDL (The Doctor's Laboratories) or similar laboratories elsewhere. They know which tests to use for conditions such as ME or CFS (chronic fatigue syndrome) and IBS (irritable bowel syndrome), which are considered by some doctors to be psychosomatic. The laboratories frequently turn up some metabolic problem which, when dealt with, helps people enormously. The precise metabolic problem often differs between patients.

CASE HISTORY: *Marie*

Marie, a scientist, had flu leading to continual fatigue (ME) at the age of 16. Between then and the age of 50 she was 'delicate', on average able to live a half life, going to bed at 7 pm and for much of weekends and holidays. At 50, on completing her 'big book' (approximately 400,000 words), she had shingles and was left an invalid. Despite her illness, she had by now published more than anyone else in her field and was awarded the Doctor of Science degree of the University of Cambridge. For the next 20 years she continued writing, mostly books, but had to spend most of her time in bed. At 70, she was hit by a lorry, which left her severely ill and able to concentrate for only about an hour a day – a grim life, particularly for someone who enjoyed work and who was trying to complete another book.

Three years later she was diagnosed with, and treated for, faulty mitochondrial ATP*. Seven months on, she is able to choose whether to write 10,000 to 12,000 words a week or to reduce her resting time to only three hours a day, with bed at 7 pm. She looks in full health, she feels well, and her health is still improving.

* The ATP test had recently been developed by Dr John McLaren Howard at a private medical facility. The test is now carried out at Acumen (see Resources). Access is by medical referral.

Prescription and recreational drugs

Another common problem in diagnosis is that the side effects of prescription[4] and recreational drugs may not be considered. One study found that 43 per cent of patients diagnosed as depressed in one practice were taking medications for some physical illness or other that can cause depression. In Jane's case none of her doctors seem to have considered that her symptoms reflected the withdrawal effects of benzodiazepines. Perhaps this is because there was no widely accepted treatment available, although taurine works for many people (see Chapters 1 and 6).

Janet was also clearly misdiagnosed. She was not questioned about using recreational drugs and was treated as a schizophrenic – although there was no evidence of any previous history of mental illness and, indeed, there have been no recurrences in the 25 years since. The UK National Schizophrenia Fellowship warns that using street drugs might make someone appear to be mentally ill for a short time, when this is not really the case.[5]

Janet should have been kept under observation until the effects of the cannabis had worn off before any diagnosis was made. Being treated with drugs for schizophrenia might well have aggravated her condition, as would the terror she felt at being locked in a mental hospital.

We are aware of many situations in which patients are prescribed medication without any physical examination or tests for underlying physical conditions being carried out first, and also many cases where problems from prescribed or recreational drugs are not considered or discussed with the patient.

CASE HISTORY: *Robin*

Robin, aged 24, had been in hospital for serious depression and psychosis and been given progressively stronger medication, including SSRIs and tricyclic antidepressants and antipsychotic drugs. It took several sessions of psychodynamic therapy for Robin to feel safe enough to disclose that he had been using 'skunk' (very strong cannabis) since he was 14 and he had become addicted. His father was often absent but even when he was at home was emotionally distant. However, Robin did have a close relationship with his mother. By the time he sought therapy he had lost interest in almost everything and spent hours alone in his room with his computer and his 'joints'. The diagnosis he had been given had persuaded him there was no point in making any effort because there was no hope and no future. In his sessions, he gradually realised that his psychosis and depression were probably related to his use of skunk. He realised that his fantasies had been side effects of this, and managed gradually to give it up. He began to reconnect with his old friends, has a new girlfriend and is working towards gaining a degree in media studies. He no longer requires prescribed medication.

Remember that in both our own cases there were particular chemical imbalances which needed to be corrected for them to be effectively cured, so try to think of anything that could be a factor in your case. If you have taken recreational drugs or have a problem with alcohol tell your doctor about this. In our cases no amount of talking therapy would have solved the problem, which was mainly related to a chemical imbalance. In other situations, for example PTSD, a specialist therapist is most likely to help while in others, for example some anxiety states, some type of talking therapy will be most helpful.

Circumstantial causes

Try not to accept drugs without diagnosis. If you have not had anxiety or depression before and you think your low mood reflects some recent major setback, ask for counselling and try to finish the course before taking pills. Most people eventually come to terms with losses and changes, and talking about situations can help. If your doctor is unable to provide counselling, seek their support in finding help yourself, privately if you can afford to pay or through a charity such as Samaritans, or a charity that offers counselling for particular situations such as bereavement or a diagnosis of cancer. Some of these are listed in the Resources section at the end of the book.

The next step

If, after a few weeks, your symptoms are still there or if no underlying physical illness is diagnosed, the next step is to discuss treatment for your anxiety or depression with your doctor. This will vary depending on the condition. With most anxiety states, talking therapies should be considered first and your GP should be able to refer you to a specialist in cognitive behavioural therapy (CBT) in the first instance. If your anxiety persists or if you have other unpleasant symptoms of depression try to persuade your doctor to obtain a diagnosis based on levels of neurotransmitters and their metabolites in a sample of urine (such tests cost about £250–£300). Remember, at the simplest level some types of depression are related to there being too little serotonin in synapses while others are related to too little noradrenaline. Only after the results of such tests are available should medication be considered. If your GP will not do this and you can afford it, it is well worth paying privately to obtain a good diagnosis and treatment plan. Laboratories that will carry out such tests are listed in the Resources section at the end of the book.

It is vital that the doctor prescribes the best drug for you, and at the correct dose, and we believe that good diagnostic tests prior to prescribing medication should be available to everyone. So, let's look at how diagnosis could be improved.

Diagnostic tests on urine and blood samples

Although they are not widely used in the UK or US, more sophisticated diagnostic tools are available that are used in other countries and in some private clinics in the UK and US.

Some laboratories use analytical methods such as HPLC (high pressure liquid chromatography) and GCMS (gas chromatography mass spectrometry) to analyse urine or blood samples to identify which neurotransmitters are too high or too low. Both types of sample have been shown by research to reflect levels of neurotransmitters in the brain.[6]

There is nothing extraordinary in determining levels of organic chemicals, especially such simple molecules as the neurotransmitters, in samples using HPLC or GCMS. Both analytical techniques use standard widely available equipment that is used by the oil and gas industry and by environmental consultants to determine levels of contaminants. Jane routinely used both HPLC and GCMS analyses for her work as an environmental geochemist and was in charge of these laboratory facilities at the British Geological Survey.

Levels of neurotransmitters – including noradrenaline, adrenaline, dopamine, serotonin and GABA – in the samples are compared with reference levels, together with the levels of neurotransmitter precursors and neurotoxins. Many different problems are indicated by different patterns of neurotransmitters identified in blood or urine samples. For example, problems with the GABA system that affected Jane are readily identified and can be treated using targeted amino acid therapy, as Jane discovered by using taurine (see page 125). The results are easy to interpret and apply and we have helped several patients to have such tests before being treated by their GP. The diagnosis for each condition is used to devise treatment based on conventional drugs but at much lower doses than usual and often in combination with amino acids. Herbal or homoeopathic treatments may also be used (see page 126).

Interestingly, a report in the 6 December 2006 issue of *Journal of Neuroscience*[7] reported that scientists at the University of Bristol have found that 'a person's sense of taste responds to changes in neurotransmitter levels. The test helped identify whether their mental health problems are with noradrenaline or serotonin.' Sweet tastes were less well identified in serotonin deficiency and improved by taking SSRIs whereas low noradrenaline levels were found to affect our sour taste. One of the psychiatrists who co-authored the report is quoted as saying 'British doctors get it right 60 per cent of the time [in the medication they prescribe]. What we're working towards hopefully is to try to find a marker so that we can tell if they've got a serotonin problem or a noradrenalin problem or both.' The researchers seem totally unaware of the work of Dr Fuad Lechin, a distinguished doctor and neuroscientist at the Central University of Venezuela Institute of Experimental Medicine, and his followers (see page 104). They appear not to have done that most essential first task of any research programme – a thorough literature survey – or they would know that a much more advanced system based on determining levels of neuro-transmitters is already available, including in private clinics in the UK!

CASE HISTORY: *Rebecca*

Rebecca was married with two children and had managed to cope with her family duties and a musical career for many years. She remembered how initially she had begun to feel low for just a few days at a time, but this low mood began to last longer and longer and increasingly took over her life. One of the most distressing symptoms was her inability to concentrate, so that her career was badly affected and finally destroyed. She was treated over a considerable period of time by her GP, who reassured her that she was not seriously ill but eventually prescribed SSRI antidepressants for her. Within days, she returned to the surgery to say how these were making matters worse, but she was persuaded to persevere. After a few weeks, she simply gave up taking them and began to feel a little better until one of her daughters had a miscarriage for the third time. Rebecca felt totally unable to cope. She was persuaded to have her neurotransmitters tested via a urine sample. The results clearly showed she was suffering from dysthymic depression, with no detectable noradrenaline but with levels of serotonin that were too high. It was recommended that she be prescribed a low dose of a noradrenaline reuptake inhibitor combined with the amino acid phenylalanine, which is converted to noradrenaline in the brain. She was able to buy and take the phenylalanine immediately, but unfortunately her GP refused to believe the results meant anything and refused to read the articles about the method of diagnosis. She was forced to go to a doctor in Harley Street to obtain the prescription for the noradrenaline reuptake inhibitor.

She also started to follow the nutritional guidelines outlined in Chapter 10, eating lots of walnuts as a good source of copper together with lots of freshly squeezed juices as a source of vitamin C to help in the synthesis of noradrenaline. She began to feel better after just a few days and after only a month said she felt her old self again, able to cope with her family responsibilities. She is now a grandmother and enjoys teaching the piano and copes well with life, although she keeps to her eating programme and takes phenylalanine if she begins to feel low.

Salivary cortisol

Salivary cortisol has been shown to be an excellent indicator of the cortisol concentration in the blood[8] and to offer a practical approach to assessing stress levels,[9] although results may be affected by psychotropic drugs. Since there is normally a marked variation in levels diurnally, the total concentration or the area under the curve is normally used, so several samples should be taken over the course of a day and measured. Factors such as age and sex, as well as physical illnesses and coping strategies, need to be taken into account. Since cortisol levels are a major indicator of psychological stress and reflect different types of depression, work to develop a standardised procedure is needed.

Brain scans

Brain scans, especially those that measure brain function, are used extensively in research into mental illness. We know, for example, that the brains of female monkeys with symptoms of depression, such as low activity levels, disruptions in hormone levels and higher heart rates, show similar results on scans to those of depressed human females,[10] and we are told that brain scans can be used to predict which antidepressants patients will respond to.[11] They are even used to check how well advertisements will work on us.[12] In practice, however, the use of brain scans in the diagnosis and treatment of mental illness is restricted almost entirely to the private sector where doctors are trained to look for the subtle changes associated with different mood disorders. Otherwise, brain scans are used in medicine almost entirely for diagnosing conditions, such as strokes and Alzheimer's, where there are clear and simple neurological changes.

Dr Daniel Amen, an eminent neurologist and Professor of Psychiatry at the University of California, and one of the pioneers of the clinical use of functional brain imaging as well as author of many famous books including *Healing Anxiety and Depression*, has suggested that symptom clusters, including those based on the Diagnostic and Statistical Manual (DSM) checklist (see page 33), have little or nothing to do with underlying brain function. He and his colleagues use scans not only to diagnose and treat illness but to monitor the brain healing in response to treatment. According to Amen, most psychiatrists do not look at brain function because imaging is not part of their tradition or training, many do not know how to read scans or what they mean.

Scans such as EEG (electroencephalogram), MRI (magnetic resonance imaging) and CT (computed tomography), which show the shape of the brain and are widely used for other medical purposes, rarely show anything wrong in patients suffering from anxiety or depression.[13] Their use has been likened to examining a car engine when it is switched off, because the problem with mental illness is usually with function, not anatomy, and in the last decade it has been recognised increasingly that anxiety and depression are not anatomical disorders but are problems of brain function.

The most powerful techniques for studying brain function are positron emission tomography (PET), which uses minute amounts of radioactivity to look at blood flow in the brain, and functional magnetic resonance imaging (fMRI), which has the advantage of not using ionising radiation. Both of these techniques are available in research centres. Single photon emission computed tomography (SPECT) is claimed to be practical and cost effective for use with patients.

SPECT involves injecting the patient with tiny amounts of a radioactive isotope in a substance readily taken up by the brain.[14] As the isotope breaks down it releases energy in the form of gamma rays that are detected by a rotating computer. The images are converted into sophisticated maps and three-dimensional images of the blood flow and metabolism in the brain, using advanced computer processing. The images can then be used to identify psychiatric and neurological illness.[15] Standard psychological tests are usually administered during the scanning process. SPECT functional brain imaging is available in many hospitals in the UK and elsewhere, although it is used mostly in diagnosing conditions such as Alzheimer's disease in the elderly, Parkinson's disease or epilepsy in children.

Interestingly Amen points out that there is no simple pattern for anxiety or depression. In some conditions certain parts of the brain are overactive and others are underactive but this differs according to the patient's illness.[16] The different patterns have been grouped into seven different clusters with different treatment regimes, all which 'light up' specific parts of the brain when certain conditions or patient mind-states are created. The Society of Nuclear Medicine has established a large database of PET scans at Yale University in the US for clinical and research use. A database of PET scans of children has been published.[17] Amen describes how patients respond to traditional therapy and medication, as well as to a host of alternatives, such as herbs, nutrients, and various other interventions after a diagnosis using SPECT.

Dr Amen nevertheless emphasises that, as with any other medical test, SPECT should be used only in the context of a patient's history and examination. It is not suitable for all patients and it is not simply a 'doctor in a box'. It requires a fundamental understanding of the brain and its workings.

There is much opposition to the use of such scans[18] but most attacks on the method have little substance and read as if they are written by people with more old-fashioned skills trying to defend the status quo. This is almost always the case with major scientific advances.

A new approach

Over the last decade scientists and doctors,[19] notably in South America and Germany, have developed an approach to depressive illness based on a fundamental understanding of neurophysiology and neurocircuitry following tests on blood and urine samples. This method of diagnosis and treatment, pioneered by Dr Fuad Lechin, is used by some private clinics in the UK.

In the case of depression four main types are recognised linked to the reactions of experimental animals to stress, described in Chapter 3, and following the identification of neurotransmitter disturbances in animals and humans. All of the conditions are described as neuro-autonomic disorders, in other words problems with the autonomic nervous system as described in Chapter 3.

Based on the work of Lechin and his co-workers and followers, four main types of depressive illness and stress are recognised:

1. Endogenous (or unipolar or major) depression
2. Dysthymic depression
3. Coping stress
4. Uncoping stress

Like Amen, Lechin and his followers acknowledge that the four types of depressive illness are difficult to distinguish clinically and that medication cannot be prescribed on the basis of symptoms alone. Treatment is aimed at correcting chemical imbalances, especially imbalances of neurotransmitters in the brain. They use only low doses of neuropharmaceutical drugs, including antidepressants, usually for a few weeks and usually in combination with other methods considered complementary in the UK (see page 148–51). Benzodiazepines are never used, because of evidence that they prevent normal sleep by suppressing rapid-eye-movement (REM) sleep and two phases of slow-wave sleep (SWS) which are needed to recover intellectual function. The four types of depressive illness are described below, together with the methods used for treating the conditions.

1. Endogenous (unipolar or major) depression is characterised by increased central noradrenaline activity and lower than normal central serotonin levels, with low plasma tryptophan and platelet serotonin. There is generally underactivity of the adrenal glands (adrenaline and cortisol) with an increased noradrenaline to adrenaline ratio. People with endogenous depression are described as having normal or even improved immunity. This model is fairly consistent with the Western model of unipolar depression except for the evidence of underactivity of the adrenal glands. Evidence that this type of depression follows a major stressful event suggests that it is an adaptation to stress.

Because endogenous depression is characterised by reduced serotonin and increased noradrenaline activity, drug treatments that involve increasing noradrenaline frequently fail because levels are already too high. According to the Lechin school, the most successful treatments for endogenous depression involve the use of drugs such as SSRIs, which reduce central noradrenaline activity by strengthening the antagonistic serotonin activity.

2. Dysthymic depression, in contrast, is characterised by low noradrenaline levels and dopamine activity but with raised plasma serotonin. The noradrenaline to adrenaline ratio is generally abnormally low when the patient is at rest, but it becomes normal (in the range 2–4) as a result of exercise. Like endogenous depression, this condition is associated with low adrenal activity and poor response to stress, with diminished activity on the HPA axis.

It is suggested that this type of depression indicates low activity of the adrenal glands and sympathetic nervous system, accompanied by increased parasympathetic activity. Dysthymic depressives are considered more likely to develop symptoms of uncoping stress than 'normal' people or those with endogenous depression.

Dysthymic depression is recognised by Western medicine but is generally described as a mild form of depression rather than a fundamentally different type of illness requiring a different type of treatment. Clearly dysthymic depression, characterised by increased serotonin and low noradrenaline levels, requires an entirely different treatment to endogenous depression, since the condition is likely to be aggravated by treatment with SSRIs. People with this condition are more likely to benefit from noradrenaline reuptake inhibitors. Unfortunately, patients with dysthymic depression are frequently diagnosed as suffering from a mild form of depression and treated with low-dose SSRIs. The dose may be increased if they do not respond.

3. Coping stress is associated with increased noradrenaline, reflected in an increased noradrenaline to adrenaline ratio, but with a reduced level of cortisol. Peaks of noradrenaline but not adrenaline or plasma cortisol occur when the person is submitted to stress, including exercise. People with this condition can develop the far more serious condition of uncoping stress if stress is repeated or prolonged.

4. Uncoping stress is closely similar to a condition known as behavioural despair in experimental animals subjected to inescapable trauma. Experiments on animals have shown that when an animal experiences a trauma it cannot control (for example, whatever path through a maze it takes, it still receives an electric shock) it simply gives up. This condition is accompanied by exhaustion of noradrenaline, which is compensated for by increased activity of the adrenal glands resulting in high levels of adrenaline and cortisol. Noradrenaline to adrenaline ratios can be as low as <1 to 2. As in dysthymic depression, there is increased activity of the parasympathetic nervous system in such patients. Levels of plasma serotonin can be high enough to damage immune function and there is often increased platelet aggregation – with an increased risk of cardiovascular disease – a feature not seen in endogenous depression. The fact that 40 to 60 per cent of those diagnosed with depression have elevated levels of stress hormones suggests that a high proportion of those diagnosed with depression are likely to be suffering from uncoping stress.

As well as noradrenaline, dopamine and serotonin levels in the brain are depleted in uncoping stress. Stress tests – including exercise, which causes the noradrenaline to adrenaline ratio to fall further – quickly give rise to side effects such as anxiety, dizziness, headache, tachycardia, abdominal pain, nausea or asthma. The condition is associated with marked sleep disorders and immunosuppression and it is suggested that, left untreated, it can lead to cardiovascular, gastro-intestinal, endocrine, immunological and other metabolic diseases, including cancer. Affected individuals with anxiety and insomnia frequently present with uncoping stress profiles.

The recommended treatment for uncoping stress, characterised by depletion in all the monoamine neurotransmitters, involves boosting central noradrenaline levels using tricyclic antidepressants, which include a noradrenaline reuptake inhibitor.

Lechin and others claim they have no failures using these treatment regimes, though this depends on the patient having been correctly diagnosed. They contrast their approach with that of typical Western medicine in which high, sometimes massive, doses of pharmaceutical drugs are administered, usually with no proper diagnosis of the type of depression that the patient is presenting with. They are particularly concerned about the use of noradrenaline reuptake inhibitors to treat endogenous depression. These drugs only work, it is claimed, if noradrenaline production in the brain is exhausted; this can take weeks or months, during which time the patient can become seriously ill.

We now work with doctors and psychiatrists who use the Lechin methods of diagnosis and treatment with considerable success. In some patients, treatment can be modified to a typical Western medical approach. For example, working with one psychiatrist we find that beta blockers, which directly target noradrenaline, can be used with SSRIs to improve the symptoms of endogenous depression – although the same treatment would make other types of depressive illness much worse. We emphasise that a diagnostic blood or urine test should always be carried out first. Such tests, available from a few select laboratories in the UK, identify not only the four types of depression but many other imbalances too, including the kind of imbalances in the GABA system that caused Jane such distress, as well as underlying problems such as low-level chronic infections.

CASE HISTORY: *Helen*

Helen was being treated for a recurrence of cancer, but despite chemotherapy and following the dietary and lifestyle advice in the Plant Programme[20] to the letter, nothing seemed to be helping. She was a pretty woman with a devoted husband and family who appeared to have everything to live for. After several sessions discussing her diet and exposure to harmful chemicals, she disclosed that she had abused alcohol since her teens. She had continued to drink, in spite of her cancer. She said she was trying to find oblivion, and did not enjoy drinking: indeed, she always drank what she described as 'cheap plonk'. It emerged that she had had a very difficult childhood, with a father who was seriously mentally ill and who had himself abused alcohol and become violent. On one occasion he had broken Helen's mother's ribs, causing distressing symptoms that Helen thought meant her mother was going to die. Helen thought she had caused the arguments and blamed herself. Over several months, Helen learned to revisit her childhood and came to understand that she was the victim, not the cause, of the problems. A few weeks after she finished chemotherapy, a urine sample was tested for neurotransmitter levels. This showed that she was suffering from uncoping stress. She had a helpful and supportive GP, who agreed to prescribe a short course of a low-dose tricyclic antidepressant, which Helen combined with the appropriate neurotransmitter precursors taken at particular times of the day. Gradually she began to feel stronger and was eventually able to stop abusing alcohol completely and her cancer disappeared. She still keeps strictly to the Plant Programme and enjoys her life to the full.

PSYCHIATRISTS, PSYCHOLOGISTS, PSYCHOTHERAPISTS, COUNSELLORS AND MIND–BODY THERAPISTS

As well as your family doctor, there are other health professionals who may be involved in helping to treat you, and it is important to understand the differences between them. If your illness does not respond to treatment and you become seriously ill, you are likely to be referred to a psychiatrist.

Psychiatrists are medically trained, with a qualification equal to an MD in the USA. The best psychiatrists, from Freud to Amen and Servan-Schreiber, will also be trained in neurology or neuroscience and understand the biology and physiology of the brain. Psychiatrists normally spend relatively short periods of contact time with patients, and their principal method of treatment is drugs.

Psychologists generally have a Bachelor's or Master's degree in psychology and in the US, and increasingly in the UK, a PhD. Clinical and counselling psychologists generally rely on the use of talking therapy to relieve distress. Psychotherapists can be trained in either psychiatry or psychology. There are many different schools of psychotherapy.

Counsellors are trained in therapies closely similar to psychotherapy, but they may not be medically trained or have an academic qualification in psychology. We discuss the talking therapies used by psychologists, psychotherapists and counsellors in Chapter 7.

There are a range of mind–body treatments now available on the National Health Service in the UK, including Eye Movement Desensitisation and Reprocessing (EMDR) for PTSD (post-traumatic stress disorder) and in some circumstances yoga and acupuncture. It is worth asking for these from your health professionals whether they work in state or private healthcare systems.

If you decide to find help privately we recommend that you ensure you find a qualified person who will normally belong to a professional body. For example, the British Psychological Society and the British Association for Counselling and Psychotherapy have an accredited-therapist service on their website, and there are similar national organisations elsewhere. If you decide to try the mind–body treatments ensure that you use an accredited specialist, for example, accredited by the British Acupuncture Council in the case of acupuncture in the UK. The professional organisations for such specialists are listed in the Resources section at the end of the book.

Seeing a psychiatrist

You are likely to be referred to a specialist psychiatrist if you are seriously ill with anxiety or depression to such an extent that it interferes with your daily life for a long period of time or if you suffer intense anxiety or depression, especially if you have suicidal thoughts. The psychiatrist should be qualified in neurology or other neuroscience concerned with the brain and its working, but many psychiatrists, unlike other medical specialists, may know relatively little about the organ they are trying to treat. Before accepting a referral to a psychiatrist, the patient or their supporter should check the qualifications of the psychiatrist with their GP and ensure that they have a qualification in neuroscience or neurology. There is simply no point in taking a car to a garage if the mechanic does not understand a modern car and there is no point in talking to psychiatrists who do not have an up-to-date scientific understanding of how the brain works. Unfortunately there are many who do not.

The psychiatrist will normally spend time talking to you and usually close family members to obtain a detailed case history and identify key symptoms. In some cases, especially in the US, patient interviews and symptom checklists are based on the standardised DSM (Diagnostic and Statistical Manual) of the American Psychiatric Association, but this is far from common practice in the UK. Diagnosis, even by specialist psychiatrists, is often made on a subjective basis. Even diagnosis made using standardised diagnostic manuals based on symptoms is unsatisfactory because, as already discussed, different mental illnesses have overlapping symptoms and can be difficult to distinguish. We know of many patients given entirely different diagnoses by different psychiatrists when they asked for a second opinion.

Ideally the psychiatrist will have access to functional brain-scanning equipment and will use methods such as those developed by Amen's group in the US to identify which parts of the brain are underactive and those which are overactive (see above). Serious mental illness requires precise diagnosis and a treatment plan based on this, especially before a treatment such as electroconvulsive therapy is considered.

A MORE HOLISTIC APPROACH

The treatment of patients with the different types of anxiety and depression diagnosed using the SPECT method of brain scanning involves the use of different types of medication, depending on which of the seven types of condition is diagnosed. Of key importance in both the Amen and Lechin approaches to the treatment of mood disorders is that drugs can be used more effectively and often in much lower doses. Nevertheless it would be helpful if their methods were standardised and cross referenced with one standard terminology.

In addition, treatment for mood disorders includes diet, supplements, exercise and social and therapeutic support – treatments which may be difficult to find in most health services. Try to persuade your doctor or psychiatrist to ensure you receive appropriate talking therapy and mind–body treatment if you have PTSD or another condition that might respond to these methods (see Chapter 7). In the UK it should also be possible, depending on your circumstances, to obtain the help of social services through your family doctor.

Bear in mind that holistic methods of treating anxiety and depression are used by world-leading psychiatrists/neuroscientists and have been shown to work, using tools ranging from brain scans to clinical trials. In the case of nutrition, leading doctors and psychiatrists have demonstrated its central importance in depression, post-natal depression and bipolar disorder using epidemiology, brain scans and case-controlled trials. It is unlikely that you will receive good advice on nutrition from mainstream health professionals, including UK National Health Service dieticians. We recommend that you follow the dietary and lifestyle advice given in Chapters 9 and 10 of this book, which we have used to help many people improve their mood and mental health.

THE IMPORTANCE OF GOOD DIAGNOSIS

At the beginning of the twenty-first century we need a science-based, holistic approach to the diagnosis and treatment of mood disorders and we believe you are entitled to ask for this. There are clearly many highly effective treatments available for treating mood disorders, especially drug treatments (discussed in the next chapter). The main problem is the lack of accurate diagnosis.

We know of people treated for years with SSRIs who it turned out were dysthymics for whom this was the worst possible treatment, and others whose treatment included SNRIs (see page 117) which made their endogenous depression worse. In these cases, patients' conditions improved rapidly once they were given the correct medication and the improvement was sustained. Treatment plans following an accurate diagnosis generally involve much smaller amounts of pharmaceuticals than are usually prescribed, combined with amino acid therapy. Herbal or homoeopathic approaches may also be used. We would prefer to try targeted amino acid therapies first (see page 125): for example we would take 5-HTP or L-tryptophan before trying SSRIs for endogenous or major depression. Amino acids are natural molecules, not ones engineered by man, and are therefore likely to have far fewer side effects. A good doctor will be aware of and know how to help you find such treatments while supporting you in making improvements to your diet and lifestyle. It might also be worth asking your doctor if he or she uses acupuncture or other mind–body treatment or if anyone in the practice does.

Overall, effort needs to be devoted to developing and standardising diagnostic techniques for mental illness to bring them to the same standards as those used for physical illnesses.

Chapter Six

The Chemical Toolkit

IN THIS CHAPTER, we first critically review some of the drugs that are the mainstays of conventional medical treatment of mood disorders and how they are used, and describe new and exciting treatments such as targeted amino acid therapy which Jane used to treat herself and which are already available in private clinics in the UK, US and elsewhere. We also discuss amino acid treatments and herbal therapies for stress, anxiety and depression that are used a great deal to treat mood disorders in continental Europe, especially Germany.

DRUG TREATMENTS

Drug treatments are now the mainstay of most conventional mental health systems and although many patients have benefited from their use, their prescription can be 'hit and miss'. Nevertheless, the introduction of drugs is rightly regarded as a major breakthrough in the treatment of mental illness, largely eliminating the use of frontal lobotomy operations and limiting the use of electroconvulsive therapy (ECT). Here we look at the main types of drug used. Our aim is to provide general information to allow you to compare treatments – it is not specific guidance on the use of particular drugs. You should always refer to your doctor or pharmacist for detailed information on mode of action, side effects and potential conflicts with other medication.

Types of drugs

There are four main groups of psychoactive drugs used in the treatment of anxiety and depression.

* Antidepressants: selective serotonin reuptake inhibitors (SSRIs), serotonin noradrenaline reuptake inhibitors (SNRIs), tricyclics, and monoamine oxidase (MAO) inhibitors.

* Mood stabilisers, such as lithium, normally used to treat bipolar disorder.

* So-called 'minor' tranquillisers, or anxiolytics, such as benzodiazepines and buspirone, which are often prescribed to help sufferers to sleep.

* Antipsychotic drugs (major tranquillisers), developed mainly to treat schizophrenia, but they can also be used to treat bipolar disorder and extreme anxiety.

In addition, beta blockers are used to treat the physical symptoms of stress.

The drugs are referred to mostly by their generic name, as brand names differ in different countries, so check with your doctor or pharmacist if you are unsure which type of medication you are taking.

All these drugs have been approved for use by the appropriate medical authority. In England and Wales, drugs and other treatments are approved for use in the NHS by the National Institute for Health and Clinical Excellence (NICE). In the US the Food and Drug Administration (FDA) approves drugs for use.

> ### General guidelines for using psychoactive drugs
>
> - You should inform your doctor of any other medication you are taking, including non-prescription drugs such as ibuprofen and aspirin, as well as herbal or homoeopathic remedies.
>
> - You should check if there are any foods you should avoid and if it is OK to drink alcohol while taking medication.
>
> - Many of the drugs used to treat anxiety and depression can cause drowsiness – always ask your doctor if you can drive or operate machinery while being treated.
>
> - Women who think they might be pregnant or are breast feeding should always tell their doctor before taking any prescribed medication.
>
> - You should never stop taking psychoactive drugs abruptly. Reduce the dose over a period of time under medical supervision.

Antidepressants

Whatever type of anxiety or depression you are suffering from, you are most likely to be offered some type of selective serotonin reuptake inhibitors. These may be offered for many other problems too, including eating disorders and even irritable bowel syndrome (IBS). We know of people who have been treated with these drugs for a considerable period of time when they were actually suffering from a physical problem that the doctor failed to diagnose, for example coeliac disease (see page 95).

Selective serotonin reuptake inhibitors (SSRIs)

Some of the latest drugs used to treat anxiety, depression and low mood include fluoxetine (Prozac), paroxetine (Seroxat), sertraline and citalopram. SSRIs are now used to treat many types of mental illness, from social anxiety to serious anxiety states such as panic attacks and panic disorder, obsessive compulsive disorder (OCD) and bulimia, as well as depression.[1] Unlike most of the earlier drugs used to treat depression, such as the MAOIs and tricyclics, these drugs were developed on the basis of a specific scientific hypothesis and are often used as an example of 'rational drug discovery' by a modern pharmaceutical industry, as distinct from 'discovery by chance'.

SSRIs have a more selective action than the older types of antidepressants. They use a molecule so similar to serotonin that it competes for reuptake, so that serotonin levels build up in synapses (see Chapter 3). It has been suggested that they may also promote the growth of new neural pathways, help prevent pro-inflammatory processes that are linked to depression and bipolar disease, and that they may also regulate carbohydrate metabolism.

SSRIs are not considered addictive in the way that benzodiazepines are, but coming off them can cause dizziness, fatigue and nausea and in serious cases delirium, so their use should be phased out rather than stopped abruptly. The main advantage of drugs in this group is the low risk of side effects, especially compared to tricyclic antidepressants – though these do sometimes occur and can include anxiety, insomnia, nausea and sexual dysfunction.

The SSRIs have recently been the focus of media attention because the side effects, notably in children and adolescents, have been shown to include agitation, aggression and suicidal tendencies. Psychiatrists and doctors are now generally advised to consider suicide risk before prescribing SSRIs, especially to the young.

Serotonin-noradrenaline reuptake inhibitors (SNRIs)

SNRIs, such as venlafaxine (Effexor), duloxetine and mirtazapine, are one of the newest classes of antidepressants that increase the level of both serotonin and noradrenaline. Increasing noradrenaline is considered to help with alertness while increasing serotonin is thought to improve mood. SNRIs are prescribed mainly for depressive illness and anxiety disorders but also for OCD, eating disorders and chronic physical pain. You may be prescribed these drugs if SSRIs do not work within a reasonable period of time. Common side effects include gastro-intestinal disturbances such as nausea and constipation, urinary retention, dry mouth, blurred vision, sedation, cardiovascular effects and sexual disturbance.

Beta blockers

In the past, beta blockers were used mainly for heart problems, including irregular or fast heartbeat, because they block the action of noradrenaline and adrenaline on the sympathetic nervous system, which mediates the 'fight or flight' response. They were also used for hypertension although this is no longer common because of concerns that some may increase susceptibility to type 2 diabetes. Beta blockers are now used to treat the symptoms of stress, for example because of social anxiety, but they can cause sleep disturbances.

An SSRI is sometimes combined with a beta blocker to further increase levels of serotonin relative to noradrenaline, especially in anxiety states.

Tricyclic antidepressants (TCAs)

Tricyclics[2] – so called because their molecular structure contains three rings of atoms – include drugs such as clomipramine, imipramine, doxepin and dothiepin (which Jane was treated with). The discovery of tricyclic antidepressants in the late 1950s was accidental in that they were found to improve mood when being tested as a treatment for Parkinson's disease. For many years they were doctors' drug of choice for treating depression but they have increasingly been replaced by SSRIs. They may still be used where insomnia is a major symptom or if other treatments fail to work.

Tricyclic antidepressants have been shown to be effective in clinical trials, with a significant improvement in more that 60 per cent of patients, compared with 30 per cent on a placebo. They are cheap and generally not addictive, although their use should be phased out rather than stopped abruptly.

Their precise mode of action is not fully understood but they are thought to work by blocking the reuptake of dopamine and noradrenaline from synapses, but some also block the reuptake of serotonin and some block only serotonin. However, they can cause unpleasant side effects, including confusion, constipation, dizziness or drowsiness, irregular heartbeat, tremors and visual disturbances.

Overdoses can be fatal and this is one of the reasons that SSRIs are now used more than TCAs.

Monoamine oxidase inhibitors (MAOIs)

This is a powerful group of antidepressants but because they can interact dangerously with some types of food or other drugs many are used only as the last line of defence in treating depression, or to treat atypical depression (see page 36). It is thought that MAOIs prevent the enzyme that normally breaks down monoamines, such as serotonin, from working and thus allow the levels of the monoamine neurotransmitters to build up at synapses in the brain, relieving the symptoms of depression.

When taken orally, MAOIs, especially older drugs of this group such as phenelzine and pargyline, can have serious side effects as they can interact badly with foods that contain high levels of tyramine (such as cheese, pickled fish or fermented substances, meat, yeast extract and even foods that contain a dopamine precursor, i.e. broad beans), causing high blood pressure.

Recently, a patch form of the MAOI drug selegiline became available in the US. Because it doesn't enter the gastro-intestinal tract and is absorbed directly into the bloodstream, thereby necessitating a lower dose, it decreases the dangers associated with MAOIs. Some other new MAOIs, such as moclobemide, are safer but may not be as effective as older types.

The most significant risk in using MAOIs is the potential interaction with herbal treatments such as St John's Wort and other prescription antidepressants and medications.

A chance discovery

In 1952, tuberculosis patients being treated with a new drug called iproniazid seemed to be making a good recovery. In fact, their tuberculosis was unaffected but their mood was improved by the drug treatment. It was later discovered that iproniazid and related drugs inhibit the activity of an enzyme called monoamine oxidase (MAO), which normally breaks down monoamines such as dopamine and noradrenaline in the brain.

Mood stabilisers

These are typically used to treat people with bipolar disorder, which is characterised by extreme mood swings. Several types of drugs are used to help to reduce variations in mood, including lithium, carbamazepine and valproate. All these drugs are generally considered to be safe, if taken as directed, and not addictive.

Lithium

The most commonly used mood stabiliser, lithium, is effective in treating 70 to 80 per cent of people. It has a very similar chemistry to sodium, the chemical element normally used to transmit electrical impulses between neurons, which may explain the way in which it helps to stabilise nerve-impulse transmission in the brain.

It generally takes two to three weeks for lithium to become most effective, and the level in the blood is usually monitored to ensure the dosage is safe but effective. Lithium was discovered to have beneficial therapeutic effects on bipolar disorder in 1949[3] but its use was vehemently opposed by conventional medicine and it took the FDA more than 30 years to approve it.

There has long been epidemiological evidence to support the importance of lithium for mental health. As long ago as the early 1970s, lithium concentrations in water in Texas were shown to correlate with levels in urine and both sets of values showed that admission rates to mental hospitals – and murders – increased when lithium levels were low.[4] The relationship between adequate lithium levels and mental and physical health has been confirmed by many other studies and it is now considered as an essential trace element by the WHO. Good dietary sources of lithium are outlined in Chapter 10.

Lithium, used in clinical doses, can cause side effects, especially in the early stages of treatment, including tremors, shaky hands, dry mouth and nausea or fatigue. In the long term it can result in weight gain.

Other mood stabilisers

Other drugs in this group include carbamazepine and valproate. Carbamazepine can take several months to take effect. Side effects include nausea and skin rashes, and blood levels need to be monitored carefully. As well as being used as a mood stabiliser it is used occasionally to treat benzodiazepine or alcohol withdrawal.

Valproate is used particularly for mania and it should start to work soon after treatment has started, although it may take a week or so to have maximum effect and the dose often needs fine adjustment. Again, blood levels should be monitored carefully. Side effects include nausea, skin rashes and weight gain.

Minor tranquillisers

The forerunners of today's so-called 'minor' tranquillisers were barbiturates, which were once widely prescribed as 'sleeping pills'. However, they caused sedation and were potentially fatal, particularly when mixed with alcohol. They were also addictive and could interfere with other treatments.

By the early 1960s chlordiazepoxide (Librium) and diazepam (Valium) had been discovered, which were to be the first of a class of drugs known collectively as benzodiazepines. Unlike barbiturates, they carried a far lower risk of overdose. They act by facilitating the activity of GABA, the most widespread and effective inhibitory receptor in the brain (see page 56).

They have many therapeutic uses and are safe and effective *in the short term* for treating a wide range of conditions, although dependence can develop in days or weeks in some people. They are used to treat anxiety, insomnia, agitation, seizures and muscle spasm and are often combined with TCAs and SSRIs at the start of treatment for depression.

Benzodiazepines work initially by helping patients to sleep. They do this by decreasing firing in the amygdala, the brain's fear centre, thereby cutting down the distribution of noradrenaline to the fore-brain. Some doctors and scientists strongly oppose the use of these drugs because they affect the normal sleep cycle, making it difficult to recover intellectual ability and hence coping ability.[5]

The side effects of benzodiazepines, especially the effects of withdrawal, are now well known and include difficulty with concentration and memory, aggression, particularly if they are combined with alcohol, rage and, in some cases, increased anxiety and suicidal thoughts. See also the box below.

Other drugs that target the GABA receptor and promote sleep, such as zopiclone, unfortunately often prove to have the same problems as benzodiazepines.

Benzodiazepines[6]

Benzodiazepines include Librium, Valium, nitrazepam, temazepam and Ativan (lorazepam). They are potent tranquillisers, introduced into the UK by pharmaceutical companies in the 1960s and 1970s but it had been confirmed by the early 1980s that long term benzodiazepine use leads to dependence in many people.

- The individual benzodiazepine addict is usually started on the drug by a GP or psychiatrist to help with anxiety, grief or stress. Doctors may repeat prescriptions for years. The drugs are also used for pre-medication before surgery or chemotherapy, and to assist alcohol and drug withdrawal.

- Benzodiazepines are among the most addictive drugs ever created, being more addictive than either heroin or cocaine. However, in the UK they are classified as Class C rather than Class A drugs.[7]

- Benzodiazepines can affect the chemistry of the brain. It has been claimed that there is no treatment for the neurochemical damage benzodiazepines cause, which continues even after you stop taking them.

- Dependency and withdrawal from benzodiazepines are often not recognised. Withdrawal can involve physical, psychological and behavioural changes when the drug is reduced or stopped. Symptoms include worry, anxiety (sometimes with panic attacks), perceptual problems, distortion of the senses, insomnia, nightmares, tachycardia, perspiration, depression and in some cases suicidal thoughts, feelings of unreality and in rare cases psychosis and seizures. Some people suffer for months and many become seriously ill and distressed.

- Withdrawal problems are commonly misdiagnosed as mental illness, and addicts are offered complicated psychological explanations of their withdrawal problems and wrongly treated with more drugs.

There is growing evidence that the brain can produce its own anti-anxiety compounds, which are released during periods of stress.[8] Some better ways of helping to deal with chronic stress and anxiety are discussed below and in Chapter 7.

Alternatives to benzodiazapines

Buspirone is an anti-anxiety drug that can be as effective as benzodiazepines although it is quite different chemically and it is not addictive. Moreover it is non-sedating. It is thought to work by interfering with the function of serotonin rather than acting at the GABA receptor. The main disadvantage is that it can take two to three weeks to take effect and it is often unsuitable for patients previously treated with benzodiazepine. It can have a range of unpleasant side effects including dizziness or lightheadedness, especially when getting up from a sitting or lying position; headache; nausea; restlessness, nervousness, or unusual excitement.[9]

Antipsychotic drugs (major tranquillisers)

Also known as major tranquillisers, antipsychotic drugs such as chlor-promazine (Largactil), trifluoperazine (Stelazine) and haloperidol (Haldol) were developed originally to calm patients before surgery and also proved highly effective in reducing the incidence of death from surgical shock. In the early 1950s they began to be used with psychiatric patients because they allowed even disturbed schizophrenic patients to live outside a psychiatric hospital. Some antipsychotic drugs used to treat illnesses such as schizophrenia are also used to treat psychotic depression and bipolar disorder, especially the manic phase. They are also prescribed for the treatment of serious anxiety disorders in the absence of psychosis and as a short-term treatment for acute agitation. These were the type of drugs used to treat Janet.

Chlorpromazine becomes concentrated in the brain stem and is secreted slowly, so that the effect on the brain is prolonged. It reduces responsiveness to external stimulation and gross motor activity without reducing motor power or co-ordination. A newer generation of such drugs, known as 'atypicals', have a wider range of action and include olanzapine (Zyprexa), risperidone (Risperdal), quetiapine (Seroquel) and clozapine (Clozaril).

Some can be given by injection every one to four weeks. Different types have different side effects. Older types can cause symptoms resembling those of Parkinson's disease: tremor, stiffness and involuntary movements. Other side effects include sedation, gastro-intestinal disturbances, dry mouth, weight gain, hormone disturbances and blood disorder. Newer drugs generally have fewer side effects, though all psychotropic drugs can have side effects in some individuals. While some cause confusion and sedation, they can also increase arousal.

NATURAL CHEMICALS

Amino acid therapy

This is the method Jane found using the Internet and used to treat her benzodiazepine withdrawal symptoms. It is also the approach used by the Lechin school to treat mental illness generally, following diagnosis of neurotransmitter imbalances in blood or urine samples.[10]

The main aims of such therapy are to provide the amino acid precursors of the neurotransmitters that are lacking in the brain. These precursors can be transported across the blood–brain barrier (whereas the neurotransmitter itself cannot). Jane treated her benzodiazepine addiction using taurine and 5-HTP, a precursor of serotonin, and has recommended it to others with alcohol or benzodiazepine addiction or abuse problems who have also found it very helpful. Other amino acid treatments can be used to increase levels of noradrenaline or dopamine or other neurotransmitters. L-tyrosine or L-phenylalanine are the precursors of noradrenaline, for example, while dopamine deficiency is usually treated with the extract of a bean called *Mucuna pruriens*, which is a rich source of 3, 4 dihydroxyphenylalanine (L-dopa for short), the precursor of dopamine. It is important to find reputable sources of amino acids because illness has been caused in the past when contaminated L-tryptophan supplements were sold over the counter. For a time it was available only on prescription but it is now available again over the counter. Clearly if your low mood or depression is related to serotonin *deficiency* L-tryptophan or its precursor 5-HTP is likely to be effective, whereas SSRIs are preferred if it is thought the problem is *insensitivity* to serotonin.[11]

The Lechin approach (see box pages 104–8) may combine the neurotransmitter precursors with pharmaceutical serotonin or noradrenaline reuptake inhibitors. Only tiny amounts of pharmaceuticals are used however, compared to the amounts used in the conventional treatment of anxiety or depression.

It is important to obtain an accurate diagnosis before using such therapies because as discussed in Chapter 3, different mental illnesses can have entirely different patterns of neurotransmitter imbalances. The assumption, which is often held by both conventional and alternative practitioners, is that any mood disorder can be helped by boosting serotonin. This can make matters worse, whether 5-HTP, L-tryptophan or SSRIs are used, because some mental illness reflects serotonin levels that are too high.

Jane prefers this method of treatment to using drugs since most of the substances used are from natural sources. One of the best ways of ensuring that the brain has all the amino acids and other substances that it needs for proper functioning is a good diet. Preparing and eating good food, especially in the company of good friends and family, can be one of the best methods of all of nurturing our emotional brain. We discuss this further in Chapter 10.

Other chemical treatments used in some private clinics include homoeopathy but this varies from patient to patient. The principles of homoeopathy are to treat like with like but at very diluted levels. Hence very low levels of a substance known to cause low mood would be used to treat depression.

Remember that using amino acids to boost levels of neurotransmitters in the brain also depends on there being adequate levels of the appropriate vitamins and minerals, as discussed in Chapter 10.

Herbal medicine

There are several groups of herbal substances that can be helpful, and it is worth remembering that some of the most powerful psychoactive drugs such as nicotine and cocaine are derived from plants. Herbal treatments are popular in central Europe, especially Germany. Many different treatments are available from professional herbalists. Here we outline some of the best-known treatments for stress, anxiety and depression.

Herbs for treating stress

The first group of herbal medicines, known as adaptogens in Russia, is used mainly to help cope in times of stress. These are thought to help us move through the usual emotional cycle that we go through if we receive a major setback, and adapt to our new circumstances. Adaptogens include *Rhodiola rosea* (Arctic root),[12] *Eleutherococcus*

(Siberian ginseng) and *Schizandra chinensis* (fruit of five flavours). Some of these can have adverse health effects (if taken by people with hypertension, for example) and we recommend that you use them only under the supervision of a trained herbalist and with your doctor's approval.

Herbs for treating anxiety

Herbs such as valerian (from which the name Valium derives) and German chamomile are helpful in treating anxiety.[13] Kava kava can also be helpful. One of the best treatments we know is oats. This used to be the treatment of choice for hyperactive children. A bowl of porridge is calming and helps restful sleep. Jane often has porridge at night before going to bed rather than in the morning. It is possible to buy herbal extracts of oats, often sold using the botannical name for oats, *Avena sativa*. Hops and passion flower may also help treat anxiety.

Herbs for treating depression

St John's Wort, a yellow-flowered perennial native to Europe, Asia and North Africa, often classed as a weed, has been widely used to treat depression for centuries.[14] The herb's Latin name, *Hypericum*, literally means 'over an apparition' because of its reputation for warding off evil spirits. The herb has been used to treat a variety of conditions since at least the time of Hippocrates but recently interest in it soared after its efficacy in treating mild to moderate depression was demonstrated. Several trials showed it to be as effective as conventional antidepressants and to have fewer side effects.[15] In 1996 a review of 23 studies published in the highly respected *British Medical Journal* showed it to be an effective treatment for both anxiety and depression and it has also been shown to be as effective as light therapy for treating seasonal affective disorder, perhaps because it increases the skin's sensitivity to sunlight.

The active compound is thought to be hypericin which can cross the blood–brain barrier and increase levels of serotonin, noradrenaline and dopamine in synapses. In other words it has a similar mode of action to that of tricyclic antidepressants such as imipramine. One study that compared St John's Wort and imipramine showed it to be equally effective but that a far smaller percentage of people suffered adverse side effects.

Despite all of its benefits you should always consult your doctor before using any form of St John's Wort, including as tea, because it can interact with other drugs such as SSRIs and warfarin and there are other contra-indications. If you are fair skinned it is important to remember that you will be at increased risk of sunburn if you are taking it.

Post-natal depression

The whole dried root of wild yam (*Dioscorea villosa*), which contains a range of plant sterols and plant-hormone precursors (progesterone and oestrogen), is used by some herbalists to treat post-natal depression. It is said to balance hormones in women and men, as well as being a natural anti-stress remedy.

Herbalists

A good herbalist will know the many other herbal treatments available for different types of mood disorder symptoms, such as sleeplessness, but we recommend that you always discuss them with your doctor before taking them. In the UK, a qualified herbalist will be a member of the National Institute of Medical Herbalists; established in 1864 it is one of the world's oldest professional bodies representing qualified herbalists.

NEW DRUGS

Because psychoactive drugs are so profitable many new drugs enter the market that are developments of existing drugs. Totally new drugs are also being developed including ones that would take effect sooner than existing antidepressants. For example, attempts to develop a drug based on ketamine, an existing drug used as an anaesthetic and as a painkiller, are underway. It has been observed that the drug can relieve depression in hours and that the relief can last for days. The mode of action of ketamine is to block an important receptor for the neurotransmitter glutamine. Unfortunately it can produce hallucinations, so efforts are under way to design a drug with ketamine's ability to alleviate depressive symptoms without its well-known side effects.[16]

It is clear that much can be done to treat mood disorders using chemical interventions but they are most effective if a meaningful diagnosis is made first. In the next chapter we tell you about some of the non-invasive methods of treatment that might help you, such as the different talking therapies and their advantages and disadvantages, and we also discuss methods based on accessing the emotional mind directly through the body.

Chapter Seven

Talking Therapies and Mind–Body Treatments

IN THE PREVIOUS CHAPTER we looked at treatments for controlling and suppressing the symptoms of depression and anxiety based on pharmaceuticals and herbal remedies. For some people such treatments, especially if they are used on the basis of improved methods of diagnosis, can provide effective relief, particularly for those already seriously ill. As we have learned, the cause might simply be a chemical imbalance that can be treated with a hormone injection or a food supplement, but for others it can be some deep-rooted emotional problem. There is a spectrum of cases where both chemical and emotional problems are involved. Indeed, we need to remember that the emotions affect brain chemistry just as brain chemistry affects the emotions. Emotional support through talking therapies might help therefore in a wide variety of cases. Most GPs are now aware of the benefits of talking therapy and some have their own 'in-house' practitioners, so it is worth talking to your doctor and asking to be recommended or referred if you think it would be helpful.

There is now a good model for the types of anxiety and depression in which there is a large emotional component, as discussed in Chapter 3, and many of the risk factors are better understood, as discussed in Chapter 4. There is much evidence that psychological talking therapies, some of them derived from the great Freud's psychoanalytical theory introduced over 100 years ago and some of them from the powerful psychological experimental findings of Pavlov, can help to identify the root causes of such illnesses. The patterns of behaviours that reinforce them can then be modified. There is also evidence from the latest neuroscience that methods based on accessing the emotional mind directly via the body can help greatly. Let us find out more about these methods, looking first at the different talking therapies that are available.

TALKING THERAPIES

There is little doubt that working with professionals skilled in the use of psychological talking therapies can help to heal our minds and develop coping strategies to help us live more fulfilling lives.[1] Indeed there is overwhelming evidence that therapies such as cognitive behavioural therapy or psychodynamic counselling can lift at least half of those affected out of their depression or chronic anxiety.[2] In England and Wales the official guidelines from the National Institute for Health and Clinical Excellence (NICE) state that 'psychological treatments should be available to all people with depression or anxiety disorders or schizophrenia, unless the problem is very mild or recent'.[2] Moreover, such therapy is found to be as effective as drugs in the short term and in the longer run to have more long-lasting effects than drugs; in the case of anxiety the official finding is that people are unlikely to relapse after therapy.[2] New evidence shows that talking therapies reduce overactivity in the part of the brain linked to OCD, as well as returning sleep patterns and serotonin levels to normal in people with depression. Evidence suggests that effective talking therapy causes improved metabolism in the brain's 'thinking areas', such as the forebrain, whereas SSRIs mostly affect non-thinking areas of the brain. This is consistent with Kandel's work on how the brain rewires itself – that the conscious mind works on the gene expression loop.[3] As we learned in the previous chapter, the best private clinics in the US use such methods to treat their patients in combination with medication. In this chapter we want to tell you about different talking therapies and whether they would be useful to you. We also want to give you some guidance on which ones to choose.

What it means to be human

In Chapter 4 we learned about the problems caused by adverse events in our early life that can make us vulnerable to depressive illness and the types of triggers that can lead to depressive illness later in life. Before we begin this section, it is worth reminding ourselves that much of our understanding of serious conditions like behavioural despair derives from experiments on animals. Although these provide good models for human mood disorders, humans are much better equipped to deal with problems than dogs, rats or even monkeys, all of which are essentially emotional, instinctive creatures. Humans, as a species, are unique in having a powerful brain that is capable of logical thought and analysis and of taking control of our other less rational unruly brains. Some of the best talking therapists will help to harness this capability to provide insights into the childhood events that made their patients vulnerable, and to understand the particular triggers and the patterns of behaviour and thought processes that these generate that can lead to anxiety and depression. This can go a long way in helping us to develop effective coping strategies to take control of the emotions and instincts in our unconscious mind that otherwise can create mental turmoil.

Understanding triggers and patterns

It is generally accepted that one of the most effective approaches in treating mood disorders is to have some form of counselling or psychotherapy in which the areas of one's life that contribute to stress, anxiety and depression can be explored in a safe non-judgemental environment. There are often significant life events that may increase or decrease stress experiences on a daily level and the way these are dealt with often reflect behaviour patterns laid down in childhood. As we learned in Chapter 3, implicit memory is central to anxiety and depression, so it is important to identify the likely problems that trigger anxiety and depression in individual patients. For example, a child who felt rejected by its parents, perhaps because of the birth of a more favoured younger sibling, is likely to overreact to real or perceived rejection as an adult whereas a child who was physically or verbally abused is likely to overreact to the slightest sign of aggression. Understanding the triggers in our lives and gaining insight into our problems can break unhelpful patterns of behaviour and greatly improve our quality of life, helping us to avoid further episodes of mental illness.

Common factors that generate emotional stress that resonate with early life experiences to precipitate anxiety and depression include:

- Changes in personal relationships, especially bereavement or loss of a close relationship through separation and divorce

- Serious family problems, marital discord and difficult relationships with lovers, friends or relatives

- Employment or career problems; loss of financial status or a serious debt burden; and physical health problems.

In addition to such major life events, we all struggle with daily problems and sometimes an apparently minor problem, such as losing something, can be the last straw and trigger feelings that life has become painful, even unbearable. The feeling that we can't cope, that we can't go on, can be intensified by all sorts of physical stressors, as discussed in Chapter 4.

Talking therapies, such as psychodynamic counselling and cognitive behavioural therapy, can help to uncover the underlying causes of anxiety and depression and develop coping strategies and ways of interpreting the feelings, making them more bearable. They are particularly effective in treating anxiety, in which spontaneous recovery is less common than with depression and in which relapse is also less likely.[4]

Here we give a brief overview of some of the better-known talking therapies and discuss how they work: 'While each approach emphasises certain aspects of human functioning and uses different therapeutic skills, it has been argued that most depend on common factors such as healing (second chance) relationships, a good fit between client and counsellor and the readiness of clients to be helped.'[5]

Sessions also depend on the training, theory, techniques and world view of therapists. When seeking help, it is important to find out what type of approach the counsellor or therapist uses, how it relates to your problem, how long therapy will take and what professional body the counsellor or therapist belongs to – and, if you are seeking help privately, how much it will cost. Bear in mind that psychotherapy is usually considerably more expensive than counselling.

A word of caution before you begin

It is important to realise that many of the talking therapies will involve you in revisiting and uncovering problems you experienced as a child, but in most cases there is no point in attacking your parents for what they did in the past because this will simply set up further cycles of stress. In some serious cases of child sexual abuse, however, it may be necessary to confront parents with the help of your therapist and discuss the issues.

The vast majority of parents do their best, but still make mistakes. There is no such thing as a perfect parent or a wonderful childhood. Therapy often highlights where things have gone wrong and can trigger resentments, but the important thing for most people is to understand, forgive and move on, remembering that forgiveness can be just as beneficial to the giver as the receiver.

As adults we can learn to see the events in a different context and, with the help of a good therapist, change our understanding of them. We cannot change our experiences, but we can change how we interpret them.

Horses for courses

There is much academic debate about the value of the different talking therapies, much of which is unhelpful if you simply want to find help. Here we try to give you simple practical advice to find the best therapy for you and your situation.

Generally, psychotherapy is most helpful where there are deep-rooted emotional problems causing serious depression. Psychody-namic counselling, which also derives from Freudian psychoanalysis, aims to identify difficult early life experiences and break the patterns they have generated that continue to cause us problems in our daily lives. It can be helpful in treating a range of problems from depression to anxiety as well as substance abuse. Cognitive behavioural therapy is aimed at training us to control our thinking by systematically examining our assumptions and beliefs and helping us to develop coping strategies. This method is highly promoted for many types of mood disorder and is particularly successful in treating anxiety, including serious conditions such as OCD. At the simplest level you might find counselling helpful; it is particularly useful in addressing low mood after a serious life-changing event such as bereavement in those previously unaffected by anxiety and depression.

Psychotherapy/counselling psychology

Psychotherapy is aimed at bringing about far-reaching, permanent changes in the patient's thinking, and tends to focus on the deep, entrenched unconscious processes and patterns which are thought to derive from our early childhood relationships and innate drives, offer-ing hope for those for whom symptom-oriented counselling offers only temporary relief. Most courses of psychotherapy continue for several months, though some shorter forms of treatment exist. Most psychotherapists and counselling psychologists have had a lengthy training and will have had to undergo their own personal therapy in order to unravel and work through unconscious conflicts and drives so that they can separate their own issues from those of the client.

Jane was helped by a wonderful psychotherapist at London's Charing Cross hospital after having her breast removed when she had breast cancer. She is still incredibly grateful for the help she was given in coming to terms with the loss of her breast. As she describes in *Your Life in Your Hands*, she remembers how her distrust of psychiatrists from observing how they had treated her father led her initially to refuse such help. The doctor involved reassured her, however, that she would not under any circumstances suggest the use of drugs or electroconvulsive therapy. She had first trained to be a surgeon but thought this was rather like being a plumber, so she had then retrained in psychiatry but thought this was simply acting as a drug pusher and was now committed to the use of talking therapies alone.

Unfortunately there are few doctors as brilliantly clever and able as Jane's psychotherapist, which is why the treatment by doctors who are also psychotherapists is so expensive and difficult to access, especially under the National Health Service in the UK or other state health care. Senior practice nurses or counsellors may now be trained in psychotherapy, however, and your doctor may be able to refer you to such a therapist for help.

Psychodynamic (Freudian) counselling (PDC)

Janet initially trained as a psychodynamic counsellor prior to becoming a chartered psychologist/psychotherapist. She has had many years of experience in helping people with a wide range of problems, including drug and alcohol abuse.

Classically this therapy involves transference, whereby the patient transfers their earlier conflicts that led to their symptoms onto the analyst. For example, someone trying to work through bad early life experiences with their father may transfer their hatred of their father onto the analyst and play them out in the talking cure. Once the early conflict is re-enacted, the analyst tries to make the patient conscious of what had been in their unconscious mind. The analyst then seeks to guide the patient to a better solution to the original conflict, ideally helping to remove the troubling symptoms.

CASE HISTORY: *Judy*

Judy needed only 12 sessions of PDC to overcome her anxiety and depression. She was a recently divorced attractive middle-aged woman. Her children had grown up and left home and she had met someone on the Internet who she felt was 'Mr Right'. She couldn't understand why she wasn't happy – she had moved into her own place and was good at her job.

Her main problem was that when she was alone in the evenings she would become frantic if her new boyfriend didn't call her. She was worried because he was younger than she was and she was terrified that he might have found someone else. She had started to drink at least one bottle of wine on nights he didn't phone to quell her anxiety and help her sleep and was afraid that this was becoming a problem.

Her father had been ten years older than her mother and used to spend most evenings at the pub, leaving her mother alone and unhappy with the children. One night, she woke up and couldn't find either of her parents. Her mother had gone to the pub to find her father and she was too small to reach the front door-knob. She remembers sitting down and sobbing and feeling totally abandoned and terrified. As a helpless child, there was nothing she could do.

This experience, deep in her unconscious which she had almost forgotten, was the key to her deep fears. While married with children, there was always someone in the house, but her recent independence and uncertainty about her relationship had triggered some deep-rooted anxieties about being alone. She was helped to revisit the feelings she had had as a frightened child left alone and realised that her interpretations and behaviour now were no longer serving any purpose. With this awareness her anxieties abated, her confidence improved, her drinking reduced and she began to feel more comfortable when alone in her house. Ironically her new boyfriend is now the one pushing for them to be together.

A fundamental belief of the psychodynamic approach continues to be that we are driven by our unconscious mind, which continues to rely on coping strategies that we adopted as children.[6] We therefore continue to repeat early patterns of feelings, thoughts and behaviour. These patterns often belong to past relationships (with mother or father or other important carer, implying that some power relationship is being brought to play). Patterns laid down in childhood, in which difficult feelings and experiences were ignored or repressed, may have served us well at the time but can lead to difficulties in adulthood. When these patterns of thought are repeated in the therapy session, they give important clues as to how relationships in the world outside the consulting room are construed. The therapist is able to bring an awareness of these dynamics to the patient and this opens up ways of resolving and changing the patterns, leading to greater freedom.

The aim of this therapy is, therefore, to help us to express ourselves freely and to find and examine the damaging negative thought processes that block more constructive thinking. The therapist will notice the silences as much as the spoken word, and will draw attention to the repetitions in behaviour patterns in our lives. The feelings (conscious or unconscious) transferred to the counsellor during the session are seen as a clue to the way we operate and see ourselves in relation to others.

Psychodynamic counselling requires that we are prepared to work towards gaining some insight or capacity to reflect on our actions in order to make maximum use of the opportunity to make fundamental change.

CASE HISTORY: *Charlotte*

When Charlotte started having counselling she was extremely nervous, she clutched the arms of the chair trying to appear calm. She was due to be married and go on honeymoon and was afraid that her anxiety was going to spoil everything and that her fiancé would change his mind about her.

She had started waking up in the night feeling so panicky she could hardly breathe. She was afraid of being a passenger in cars or on buses or planes and she needed to be near the exit in cafes, bars or restaurants and had begun to wish she didn't have to go on holiday or get married.

She was the eldest of three children. Her parents had divorced when she was young and she lived with her mother. They were permanently on the move, sometimes staying with friends, often in tiny rooms as her mother tried desperately to find a new husband. Charlotte remembers crying at night and waking up, not knowing where she was or where her mother was.

During therapy she revisited her childhood and also learned relaxation techniques. She realised that she had felt extremely angry as a child but that she hadn't felt able to express her rage for fear of losing her mother. She was currently in a situation in which she was loved and secure but was afraid to allow herself to relax and believe that she could be cared for because she was unused to trusting anyone. Her repressed emotions had been making her life unbearable.

She gradually relaxed and two or three months after the start of therapy she began to feel better and to sleep through the night. Eventually, by understanding how her past was affecting her, she grew more confident and was able to discuss her feelings and needs with her fiancé, thus breaking the pattern of repressing her emotions established in childhood.

Cognitive behavioural therapy

Aaron Beck's cognitive theory of emotional states[7] is closely linked to problems in the development of parent–child relationships. Cognitive theory holds that certain negative beliefs about ourselves, other people and events develop and are encoded in our brains from an early age until they become automatic. Typically, these include the person's dysfunctional view of themselves as defective and worthless, of the outside world as hostile and threatening and of the future with the conviction that their illness will continue for ever. Such beliefs, although they are often initiated by problems in the early parent–child relationship, become entrenched as a result of later losses and traumas, especially those that resonate with our early life experiences. In effect, it is thought that a negative feedback system becomes established in the minds of patients.

Beck discounted the idea that feelings and behaviour are simply under the control of negative forces in the unconscious mind that must be penetrated by psychoanalysis. He proposed that the patient is, in principle, able to understand and help deal with their condition. The aim of cognitive behavioural therapy (CBT) is to help the patient to unravel distortions in thinking and learn to develop more rational problem-solving approaches. It attempts to train the patient to use and develop their rational human brain rather than be overwhelmed by turmoil in their emotional mammalian and instinctive reptilian brains.

Generally, CBT is about eliminating or reducing distressing

behaviour and is not concerned with alleged causes or global personality changes. Behaviour therapy stems from psychological science in the 1920s and clinical psychology in the 1950s, which was based on accurate observations of problematic behaviour, generating testable theories and producing effective remedies. Its origins have been attributed to the findings of Pavlov,[8] who discovered that it was possible to condition or train dogs to behave in different ways using reward-based methods. This is particularly interesting because, as we learned in Chapter 3, it is our emotional mind that causes many of the symptoms of anxiety and depression. You may have seen television programmes showing how dogs can be retrained, even ones that have been badly abused in the past. Eric Kandel, the Nobel prizewinning neuroscientist, has demonstrated how the brain changes its neural circuitry as an animal changes its behaviour. Learning always involves the same neurons; the differences in learning reflect the establishment of new connections between neurons.[9]

One of the ways that CBT is thought to work is by helping the prefrontal cortex of the human brain take better control of the amygdala, and this has been confirmed using brain scans. These show high levels of frontal activity when there is a tug of war between the depression and the patient's attempts to self correct. When the attempt succeeded the frontal lobes could relax and scans showed reduced activity.[10, 12]

Cognitive behavioural therapy is now one of the most widely available talking therapies in England and Wales, following its endorsement by NICE. It is considered to be based on sound scientific principles derived from experimental psychology and has been shown to be effective in randomised controlled clinical trials where one group of patients were treated with CBT and the others just chatted to a therapist without undergoing therapy or counselling. Cognitive behavioural therapy is particularly successful in treating serious anxiety states, such as generalised anxiety disorder (GAD) or obsessive compulsive disorder (OCD).[11]

Again Jane was helped greatly by CBT when she first had cancer. She found it particularly helpful in preventing her mind constructing frightening scenarios for the future and learned to stop building what she called 'huge worry castles based on a few bricks'. Although perhaps costly to the NHS at the time, Jane's psychotherapy and CBT had no negative after effects and she was able to return to work quickly and to continue to work effectively. Compare this with the human and financial costs of the after effects of the benzodiazepines she was treated with when her cancer returned five years later.

CASE HISTORY: *James*

James had been prescribed antidepressants by his GP because he was suffering from anxiety and was unable to sleep. During his first session he was incredibly tense and rigid and appeared not to be breathing even when he was talking.

He was lonely, over-burdened with responsibility and suffering from depression and anxiety. He had recently split up with his girl-friend and was working out of his rented flat. He was having difficulty getting up in the mornings but couldn't go back to sleep and had started to panic and hyperventilate. His symptoms were beginning to disrupt his life.

During his CBT sessions he was helped briefly to explore his child-hood. He had come from a high-achieving family but the pressure he was under now seemed to be self-imposed. This combined with money worries and his isolation was causing him acute distress.

He was helped to understand the interaction of the mind and body, especially the effects of the sympathetic nervous system. He was then taught to find a comfortable place to sit and relax and to think of a sit-uation likely to cause him to panic. He was told to note the first sen-sation, whether it was his heart pounding or his palms sweating. James identified his first physical symptom as a tightening of the chest, fol-lowed by a racing heart and then sweaty palms until a full-blown panic attack had developed.

He learned with therapy to notice the first symptom and then to train himself to avoid going into a full-blown panic attack by con-sciously relaxing, including by deep diaphragm breathing. He was encouraged to draw a line down the middle of a piece of paper and to write down his physical symptoms on the left hand side and his thoughts on the right hand side, and then to draw lines between the two to see the connections. In the case of panic attacks, the interaction between body and the emotional mind can be extremely quick. Future panic attacks can be prevented by learning to understand and control the physical symptoms associated with them.

James has also restructured his day. He now takes his lap-top to a coffee bar in the morning when he feels at his worst and does simple administrative tasks. He does more difficult work from home in the afternoon when he feels less anxious. His symptoms have improved considerably as his control over his life has increased. He also realises that he was too rigid in his belief that he needed so many hours' sleep in order to function and is sleeping much better now. He managed gradually to come off the antidepressants he was taking.

CASE HISTORY: *Amy*

Amy was a pretty young woman in her early twenties who had had to abandon her A level examinations two years earlier because of her addicton to drugs. She had begun smoking when she was 11, was binge drinking by the time she was 13 and had become addicted to skunk (strong cannabis) soon afterwards.

She was the eldest daughter of three children. Her parents were both successful professionals but her mother had stayed at home to be with her children when they were small. Amy remembers always being under pressure to do well at school to please her parents, especially her mother, but unfortunately she had had undiagnosed dyslexia for years as a child. She vividly remembered being told how stupid she was by her teachers in front of her friends and how humiliated this made her feel and how she always felt her parents were disappointed in her.

Eventually, after being diagnosed with dyslexia when she entered secondary school at 11 and being given appropriate help, she had done well and obtained seven good GSCE passes in spite of her substance abuse. She now desperately wanted to escape her drug addiction and do something useful with her life.

She was helped to see that her problems were mainly social anxiety and fear of humiliation because of the treatment she had received from her teachers as a child. She had taken alcohol, nicotine and skunk because initially they had helped to ease her anxiety.

In 12 sessions she was taken through an imaginary series of progressively more challenging social situations and taught to analyse her thoughts, feelings and reactions. She learned new coping strategies and as her confidence grew she had hypnotherapy and acupuncture to help deal with her substance abuse. She was able to return to her studies and is now at university.

Counselling

Counselling is one of the simplest but most effective talking therapies. It is generally offered to those suffering from addiction, anxiety, depression, bereavement, relationship difficulties, life crises and traumas. It is also used to teach relaxation techniques, assertiveness and methods of coping with problems and stress, and how to become more fulfilled through greater awareness generally.

A key aspect of counselling, where it differs from normal conversation, is that it offers the chance to be listened to unemotionally and without judgement, and it provides a safe environment in which to express concerns and emotions.

Although it is unlikely that you will be given direct advice, it is often helpful to be allowed the time to give voice to and reflect on some of the troublesome areas of your life. A counsellor will attempt to gain insights into the nature of your problems in a confidential, non-judgemental way – something that may not be possible when you talk to family members or friends who are personally involved in your life. They will also help you to develop appropriate changes in your thinking and behaviour and to examine alternative interpretations and strategies. Counselling may involve one session a week for a few weeks or longer. Most counsellors have a diploma or higher qualification and belong to a professional body. In the UK they should be members of the BACP (British Association of Counselling Practitioners). We think counselling is particularly suitable if you have not previously suffered from anxiety or depression but something has happened that seriously affects the fabric of your life, such as a diagnosis of cancer or the breakdown of a marriage.

CASE HISTORY: Fay

Fay was desperately depressed. She had had a happy uneventful youth and had been a model in her early twenties but she had given this up when she married. She had been happily married with a devoted husband who worked as an accountant and her two young children were both at school when she decided to take on a few modelling jobs. One evening she and some friends went out for a drink after she had finished work. She was 'chatted up' – in her words – by a gorgeous charming man called Kevin and he asked her out. She began to see him more and more, often telling lies to her husband to cover her tracks. Eventually she and her two children left to live with Kevin. Soon after Fay remarried it became clear that her new husband resented any time or attention she gave to her young sons and this started to cause rows. Kevin started staying out in the evenings and she could never contact him. They were always short of money and eventually to her horror she discovered he had run up enormous gambling debts and there was little money left in their accounts. They divorced but by this time her children had grown up and were married and living a long way away. It was understandable that she was depressed.

Fay was referred to a counsellor by her excellent family doctor. Over 12 sessions she explored her mistakes and her regrets and learned to come to terms with them. Her counsellor gave her the support and confidence she needed to find new work that she finds satisfying, to rebuild her relationship with her children and to develop new interests and friends. She was also directed to sources of help to ease her money worries. This is a much better approach to helping people with real life problems than simply giving out pills.

CASE HISTORY: Elinor

Elinor had worked as a fund manager in the city of London for most of her career. By the time she was 48 her children had left home to go to university and she had begun to feel low and to have dreadful panic attacks. She saw a counsellor privately and eventually realised how unhappy and unfulfilled she felt and that this feeling mostly centred on her work. While her children had been at home this had not mattered. She thought carefully what she would really like to do with the rest of her life. She talked things through with her family and decided to do a degree in environmental science and found that this was something she really enjoyed. She went on to do a PhD at a leading research university into the relationship between an unusual type of cancer of the bile duct and pesticides and now has her own private practice as an environmental consultant. Her depression and panic attacks no longer trouble her.

Person-centred counselling

Carl Rogers (1902–87)[12] founded this approach in the belief that all individuals have the potential to flourish in conditions which are supportive, trusting and respectful, and that these conditions enable us to thrive and develop socially responsible behaviour. Person-centred counselling has a worldwide following and is widely accepted as the foundation of positive relationships.

Rogers believed that problems arise when we receive negative feedback or are valued only as long as we conform to certain conditions. To protect ourselves, we 'distort' or 'deny' negative experiences, selectively taking out some parts of what is happening and leaving out others completely. In our attempts to suppress what we cannot consciously bear, we create internal splits, but self-protection can become self-oppression and even self-destruction, leading to anxiety, confusion, depression and breakdown.

The aim of person-centred counselling is to offer the necessary conditions to allow splits to be healed and to help us to allow feelings, thoughts and perceptions to be absorbed rather than split off.

Integrative counselling

Some practitioners take the view that no single approach works for every client in every situation and the term 'integrative counselling' is used to describe the use of two or more therapies. The approach used might combine psychodynamic with person-centred counselling, for example, or with CBT.

Help for the family

Sometimes the whole family may need help in getting to the roots of a problem which may be apparent in the illness of one or more individuals. One method that is used is to talk first to the individuals concerned and help them to analyse and express their difficulties and feelings. Eventually the therapists will facilitate meetings in which individual family members are encouraged to communicate their problems as simply and unemotionally as possible without assigning blame, which can provoke aggression. Hearing others' pain expressed in this way can help the whole family identify the problems and work on developing solutions.

CASE HISTORY: *Luke*

Luke was a good-looking man in his thirties who worked in marketing. He was seriously depressed and medication had failed to help him. He had always lived with his father and stepmother and as a child had not been allowed to meet his real mother. As an adult he was strongly discouraged from doing so. He believed he had inherited his difficulties from his mother who had always been portrayed to him as a rather uncaring ephemeral person who had simply abandoned him because she cared about her career more than him. He had very low self-esteem, which he attributed to his mother never having cared about him.

In interviewing individual members of the family it soon became clear that the problem centred on Luke's stepmother, Kath. She was the only child of a couple who had stayed together despite the father indulging in a series of affairs with women much more physically attractive than her mother. Throughout her childhood she had thought that her parents' marriage might break up at any point and was deeply insecure. When she met Luke's father, John, she was determined to hold on to him but there was a problem – Luke. She knew Luke's father would never give him up but she could not bear her new husband and his son to have contact with his ex-wife who she felt was much more attractive and clever than she was. She was sure that John would want to go back to her despite the fact she had remarried.

John was too weak a person to deal with Kath and he found it easier to give in to her and her demands. At Kath's insistence every type of trick and manipulation was used to gain control of Luke and prevent his mother seeing him and, of course, all the blame had to be put on his real mother. On one occasion when John's sister, Samantha, went to see Luke's real mother who, of course, begged for help in seeing her son, Kath was furious and John backed her up. Samantha was driven out of the family but of course Luke could not be told the real reason for this and was told that his aunt had left the family because she was offended because John had said she was anorexic (Samantha was an extremely pretty woman with a great figure).

In therapy Kath learned to understand her role in the situation and was helped to address her own problems. She was given psychodynamic therapy to help her understand the roots of her destructive behaviour and was eventually able to take part in family therapy sessions. The rest of the family learned to recognise Kath's controlling behaviours and to develop coping strategies. Luke never contacted his real mother but he now understands that she did love him but had been driven away by overwhelming problems that she could not deal with. He has overcome his depression but still goes for counselling.

Choosing the best therapist for you

When choosing a therapist, it is a good idea to think carefully about the type of approach that might suit you. This will obviously depend on the extent of your problems and the severity of your anxiety or depression. Bear in mind that psychotherapy can be expensive if the therapist is a doctor, it can take a long time and there is usually a long waiting list. If your treatment is funded by the National Health Service, it is likely that your GP or psychiatrist will influence the type of treatment you are offered. Cognitive behavioual therapy is currently favoured by most healthcare systems because it achieves results after a relatively short course of treatment and randomised clinical trials have proved its efficacy for many types of problem. If you are paying privately we recommend that you actually meet two or three therapists face to face and make a decision based on how you feel about the meeting and which one you feel will benefit you most. This is not necessarily the one you like most, but the one you feel will be best able to understand and help you.

HEALING THE EMOTIONAL BRAIN THROUGH THE BODY

At the University of Pittsburgh in the US, which is noted for its excellence in psychiatric medicine, research is being carried out into relieving stress, anxiety and depression using healing methods other than drugs or talking therapies. The main aim of such methods is to reprogramme the emotional brain so that it adapts to the present rather than continually reacting to past adverse experiences. The methods used act via the body to influence the emotional brain directly rather than using methods that depend on language, reason and talking, which are the province of the human brain.

The distinguished neuroscientist and psychiatrist Dr David Servan-Schreiber has described several methods that effectively short circuit the logical human brain that is reached by language and access the emotional brain directly through the body. These methods include eye movement desensitisation and reprocessing or EMDR and heart rate coherence training. We can, he suggests, mobilise intrinsic physiological rhythms such as eye movements associated with dreams or natural variations in heart rate to help calm our emotional brains. Before we examine these new methods let us first look briefly at some traditional methods that help calm our emotional minds via the body, such as acupuncture, yoga or other types of physical exercise. An important aim of all these methods is to establish balance between our emotional intuitive brain and our logical human brain and there is increasingly strong scientific evidence, including from brain scans, that they are effective.[13] Mind–body methods also help to balance the sympathetic and parasympathetic nervous systems.

Acupuncture, acupressure and shiatsu

Traditional Chinese medicine regards emotional and physical illnesses as an imbalance in the circulation of energy or 'life force' known as qi. Qi is believed to circulate through the body via 12 meridians which form a continuous pathway through limbs, trunk and head. Acupuncture holds that the body can be stimulated to correct its energy flow and balance by inserting a fine disposable needle or otherwise stimulating the acupuncture points. More than 350 acupuncture points have been defined on the meridians and others lie outside.[14]

One of the fundamental concepts of acupuncture is that health reflects the balance of two opposite forces, Yin and Yang, and many diseases, not just mental illness, are considered to represent disturbances or disharmony as a result of blockage or deficiency of energy in one of the forces. Yin can be considered to equate to femininity, gentleness and passivity while Yang represents aggression and masculinity, equivalent in many ways to the emotional brain and human brains respectively. Some Chinese medical practitioners equate Yin with the parasympathetic nervous system and Yang with the sympathetic nervous system. Traditionally in China three additional ways are used to regenerate qi along with acupuncture – meditation, nutrition and medicinal herbs – but acupuncture is considered the most direct.

Diagnosis is important and a traditional acupuncturist will take a full case history and ask about predisposing factors. They will often explore the personality to help to understand the individual's balance of Yin and Yang. Traditionally examination will also include an inspection of the tongue – a red tip is taken to indicate acute emotional distress – feeling the pulses and in some cases palpation of the abdomen and a search for tender sites. Anywhere between one and 12 points may be stimulated and treatment is usually painless and bloodless, although there can be an unusual aching sensation afterwards. Following sessions many people describe sensations of calm and relaxation similar to those that follow intense physical effort.

Acupuncture is the oldest documented medical procedure in use today, with records of its use dating back over 5,000 years. It was recognised by the World Health Organisation in 1978 and is now accepted by the medical establishment as effective, beyond the placebo effect, not only for anxiety, depression and insomnia but also for many physical conditions.[14] The fact that it can be used effectively to treat animals, including anaesthetising them, adds to its credibility. Importantly it has been shown to cause neurotransmitters such as serotonin and endorphins to be released in the brain and it has been shown in studies carried out at Harvard to have beneficial effects on the brain using functional brain scans. Acupuncture appears to access and act on the emotional brain directly and to block the parts of the emotional brain responsible for emotional pain and anxiety.

It is highly recommended for the treatment of mental illness by distinguished doctors such as David Servan-Schreiber. There are relatively few risks or side effects from such treatments although sometimes patients are warned not to drive machines or operate machinery for a time after sessions because of drowsiness. Once again we recommend you discuss treatment with your doctor first.

Acupressure, laser, ultrasound and electrical stimulation (electro acupuncture) may be used to stimulate points instead. The Japanese form of acupressure, shiatsu, is usually applied using the fingers, hands or elbows while the Chinese version, *tui na*, can involve pulling and rubbing.

Some doctors now offer acupuncture. Jane's new GP in London practises acupuncture. Recently he successfully treated her daughter for repetitive strain injury (RSI) in just one session. We also know many patients whose serious mood disorders have been helped by acupuncture. Look at websites of organisations such as the British Acupuncture Council to find a qualified practitioner, if your medical practice doesn't offer this kind of treatment.

CASE HISTORY: *John*

John was a highly successful business man. He had been prescribed benzodiazepine sleeping tablets but had also taken to suppressing his worries with whisky. He sought help when he realised that he felt increasingly anxious and became aware that he appeared angry and aggressive to his colleagues. He was persuaded to try acupuncture. After taking a full history of his problems the acupuncturist explained to John that he had far too much Yang and far too little Yin in his life. He was given several sessions as well as advice on diet and lifestyle. He improved steadily over the few months he was treated and despite being highly sceptical initially now attends an acupuncture session every week.

Reflexology

Many people with stress, anxiety and depression benefit from reflexology, whereby manual pressure is applied to specific areas of the feet, or sometimes the hand or ears, which are believed to correspond to areas of the body in order to relieve stress. The method is depicted on Egyptian papyri from 2500 BC and is also thought to have been used by the Chinese and by North American Indians. Modern reflexology dates from the work of Dr William Fitzgerald, who learned the technique in the early twentieth century and used it mainly for pain relief in his patients. The only risk is if too much pressure is applied to patients with bone or joint problems in their hands or feet. Moreover, it should not be relied upon for diagnosis.

Biofeedback methods

Methods of obtaining mental calm by controlling physiological responses, such as heart rate and breathing, have long been part of traditional Eastern treatments such as meditation and yoga. In the West researchers in the 1960s demonstrated that methods based on modification of heartbeat using biofeedback methods induced a state of deep relaxation and mental clarity.[15]

Such methods can be especially helpful in the treatment of anxiety and panic attacks. They work by sending signals to our older emotional brain that all is well, thereby breaking the vicious circle whereby physiological symptoms of stress and distress feed our anxiety further.

Reaching to the heart

Some of the most powerful biofeedback techniques involve psychophysiological regulation of the heart, the activity of which is closely related to that of our emotional brain. Dr Servan-Schreiber sees the heart as the main bridge between our emotional brain and body on the one hand and our logical human mind on the other. One of the most powerful methods, known as Heart Coherence, draws upon the traditional techniques of yoga and meditation, and was first described by the physicist Dan Winter. Initially patients are taught to train their thoughts inwards, setting aside worries for a time. They are advised to take deep slow breaths to stimulate the parasympathetic nervous system, concentrating especially on the out breath as in yoga. But in this case rather than focusing on the breath attention is focused on the heart and patients are asked to imagine that they are breathing through their hearts.

Next they are asked to visualise their hearts being nourished and fed with the oxygen with each in breath and it being cleansed, detoxified and set free with each out breath and to see their heart being able to work at its own pace without outside pressures of any kind. The third stage involves focusing on situations that involve love or gratitude, for example, that involve children or a pet or even a peaceful natural scene such as a beach or beautiful countryside. Coherence is shown to be established by feelings of lightness and warmth and the patient may begin to smile. Establishing coherence sends a clear signal to our emotional brains via our hearts that all is well. Achieving this state gives us access to balanced information both from our emotional intuitive brain and to the logical cognitive thoughts of the human brain so we are then much better able to deal with our problems.

Some therapists specialise in training people in heart coherence and will have computer-based methods of allowing patients to visualise changes in heart function but in most cases people can train themselves. Equipment for monitoring heartbeat and blood pressure is readily available, and this can be used initially to monitor and feed back information to help patients learn to regulate their heartbeat and blood pressure, but with time and practise they can achieve coherence without measurement. Patients are advised to practise heart coherence for 15 to 20 minutes every day.

Interestingly it has been found that chanting mantras or other repetitive texts such as reciting the rosary helps to establish coherence. In some people praying helps.[16]

In addition to improved mental health, reflected by a fall in levels of circulating cortisol, such methods can help to decrease blood pressure and improve other physiological indicators of health such as our immune response.

Other biofeedback methods

Any physiological response that can be measured can be used for biofeedback methods of treatment. Those most commonly used include those that monitor the electrical activity of the brain (EEG), skin temperature, muscle tension or electromyography, blood galvanic skin resistance (GSR) or electrodermal resistance (EDR), blood pressure, respiratory rate and blood flow. The information is presented to the patient as a continuous auditory or visual signal.

Biofeedback is often used in conjunction with CBT, relaxation and stress management training. All methods are considered to act directly on the emotional brain, improving the control of the HPA axis and the autonomic nervous system. It is simple to use and widely available from psychologists and other therapists and can be learned at home using pulse rate or blood pressure, for example.

Breathing

Anyone who has learned to do yoga will know of the importance of breathing correctly. Unfortunately many of us take lots of little fast shallow breaths especially when we are upset or stressed, which can mean that we have too little carbon dioxide in the blood. The high proportion of oxygen may equip us for fight or flight but it does not help us to feel calm and in control. Indeed some people admitted to hospital suffering from intense panic attacks are simply supervised while they breathe into a paper bag to increase the carbon dioxide in their blood. With practise we can all learn to breathe properly and this means breathing with the diaphragm.

To do this first make sure that the phone or doorbell won't ring and you may wish to darken the room. Then lie on your back and place your hands, palm down, just below your navel and breathe deeply so that you can feel your hands rising with each in breath and falling with each out breath. This means you are involving your diaphragm and breathing with all your lungs not just part of them. Just doing this can make you feel much more relaxed and in control. You can then begin to systematically relax each part of the body beginning with the feet and ending with the scalp, ensuring the jaw is not clenched, repeating the process until you feel totally relaxed and in control. Jane used this simple method of relaxing and accessing her emotional brain for 20 minutes three times a day when she had cancer. She combined it with visualising herself taking a walk along a beautiful beach or in a garden.

A method called AWARE also involves breathing.[17] After an Activating event, sufferers are trained to Watch, rather than react, and scale their anxiety or panic from one to ten; to use Arousal reduction by using self-appreciation; to slow their Respiration by prolonging their out breath; and finally to Enjoy their body settling down. This method is particularly helpful in learning to deal with panic attacks.

Breathing methods are simple to learn and apply alone or they can be used by therapists to help their patients.

The eyes have it

Post-traumatic stress disorder (PTSD) is a serious anxiety state caused by what some psychiatrists regard as a serious scar in the emotional brain that continues to generate unpleasant feelings and sensations long after the incident that generated the scar is over. It can be triggered after being involved in a serious incident such as a car accident or even the sudden unexpected breakdown of a relationship or witnessing a distressing scene, for example after a bomb attack or military exercise. Often sufferers experience unpleasant flashbacks and nightmares. The symptoms of PTSD were clearly described by sufferers after the Holocaust and following military conflicts such as the Vietnam War or the Gulf War. Functional brain scans made while patients are helped to revisit the original traumatic event are distinctive. They clearly show that the amygdala is activated as well as the visual cortex as if the patients are looking at a photograph. Interestingly, the part of the prefrontal cortex responsible for language is deactivated explaining why no words can express what sufferers are feeling.

PTSD has always been regarded as difficult to treat because the logical brain and appropriate thoughts tend to pull in a different direction from the left-over emotions of the trauma. In fact talking about the problem can aggravate the symptoms so that talking therapies are unlikely to help. Moreover medication has been found to be an unsatisfactory method of treatment.

Eye Movement Desensitisation and Reprocessing (EMDR),[18] a therapy which involves moving the eyes back and forward to imitate rapid eye movement (REM) sleep while talking through the traumatic event/s that caused the problem has been found especially helpful in treating such patients. In the US the method is widely recognised as the treatment of choice for PTSD and it has also been demonstrated to be of value in easing the emotional pain of distressing childhood memories and to be of value in treating anxiety disorders, including phobias.[19]

The method, first developed by Francine Shapiro,[20] depends on using the brain's own information processing system which is normally used when we are dreaming, as indicated by REM sleep. The work of the brain in sifting and storing information has been described as the 'psychological digestion' process by Dr David Servan-Schreiber and was described by Freud as grief work. It is this system that usually allows us to come to terms with traumas after a period of time. Sometimes, however, our ability to come to terms with traumas can be overwhelmed because they are just too painful. In that case the trauma can become locked into the emotional brain unchanged and take on a life of its own with its own neural network that can be reactivated by the smallest reminder of the original traumatic event. The success of EMDR is thought to be because it stimulates the brain's adaptive information processing system to metabolise the memory of the trauma, thereby allowing the emotional mind to heal. In the US, this treatment has been extended to a host of other conditions, including depression, eating disorders, schizophrenia and psychological stress associated with cancer. There is some dispute as to whether it is more effective than cognitive behavioural therapy, combined with repeated exposure to the stimuli that trigger PTSD.[21]

During treatment, patients are asked to follow with their eyes their therapist's hand moving backwards and forwards until their eyes are showing similar movements to those seen in REM sleep. They are then asked to visualise the situation in which their trauma occurred, all the time following the therapist's hand movements. In some cases a dramatic improvement in the patient's demeanour is apparent as the scar in their emotional brain heals; in some cases this requires just one session of therapy.

The method should be used only by highly trained therapists, who can provide a caring environment in which the patient can revisit their pain because patients may initially suffer intense psychological and physiological symptoms as they visualise the situation at the root of their problems.

CASE HISTORY: George

George is a sensitive, highly intelligent man who had spent most of his life working as a university lecturer teaching twentieth-century history. In his late teens and early twenties he had done his national service with the British Army in the Kenya of the 1950s. Unfortunately he and his fellow soldiers had come across a scene of 'utter carnage' following an attack by Mao Mao terrorists on a farm in the Rift Valley. He always avoided describing what he had witnessed but the scene was burned into his memory and had caused him untold misery for more than 50 years. His wife described how he would wake up screaming after reliving the event in a nightmare or suddenly start sweating and shaking uncontrollably if something triggered the memory of that terrible day. For years he had taken various types of antidepressants and sleeping tablets but nothing touched the scar in his brain. When we first told him about EMDR he was not very interested and thought that after more than 50 years it was unlikely to help. Finally he agreed he had nothing to lose and persuaded his GP to send him for treatment. It took four sessions but finally the memory was dealt with. He can still remember the incident but it no longer causes him the intense emotional and physiological symptoms that he used to suffer in flashbacks.

Habituation and virtual-world therapy

The aim of this treatment is to make the response to a stimulus, such as fear of flying or of spiders, diminish with repeated exposure. Habituation has traditionally been used to help people with a wide range of panic disorders and phobias and involves progressively increasing exposure to the source of fear. Clinicians are now increasingly replacing reality with 3D computer simulations. Such treatment requires no travel or complicated arrangements and is found to trigger less fear, so that the patient is more likely to complete the course of treatment. Virtual-reality technologies are also being used to help fight post-traumatic stress disorder, eating disorders and OCD. The new computer-based technologies are often used with CBT to improve the behaviour component of the therapy and are thought to offer an effective low-cost method for treating a wide range of mental illness.[22]

MIND–BODY EXERCISE

Several types of exercise are thought to strengthen and enhance body and mind, including t'ai chi and yoga.

T'ai chi

T'ai chi[23] has a long history in China and is still widely practised there. It is not uncommon to walk through a park in China, Japan or Korea and see people doing their t'ai chi exercises there. Indeed, if someone is giving a boring paper at a conference, instead of going to sleep people may leave their seats and start practising t'ai chi in the aisles. Jane has seen this happen during conferences in Hong Kong and Korea.

The various types of t'ai chi comprise a series of postures linked by gentle movements thought to balance the two opposing life forces fundamental to Chinese philosophy, Yin, the reflective female force and Yang, the male creative force.

The alternating movements and postures of t'ai chi are thought to enhance inner harmony and emotional balance. T'ai chi also strengthens the muscles and the cardiovascular and nervous systems, producing better co-ordination and balance. It is recommended for stress, anxiety, depression and fatigue although it is generally regarded as an adjunct to some other treatment, not as an alternative treatment in itself. T'ai chi is usually taught in classes of five to ten people. Daily practice is best and the early morning is thought to be the ideal time of day.

Yoga

The word 'yoga', derived from Sanskrit, the classical language of ancient India, means oneness, expressing the belief that the individual is part of the universal whole.[24] The later word yoke may have similar roots and some writers use this to suggest that the purpose of yoga is to harmonise body and mind. Yoga developed in the East alongside Hinduism, Buddhism and Jainism; indeed the Buddha and Mahavira, the founder of modern Jainism, were both practitioners. Yoga was first taken into the Middle East by early Muslims. It is associated more with independent thinkers than any particular religion, however.

Yoga is believed to have developed on the Indian subcontinent more than 4,000 years ago. British administrators posted to India during the time of the Raj became the first yoga teachers in the West although the method was derided initially. It gained in popularity after the violinist Yehudi Menuhin was successfully treated for a frozen shoulder by a famous yogi known as B.K.S. Iyengar in the 1950s and its popularity grew following the Beatles' interest in Indian culture in the 1960s.

Yoga uses gentle exercises, frequently involving stretches, postures or poses (asanas), breath control and meditation to increase awareness of the body and still the mind. Most yogis and teachers stress, however, that yoga is more than simply a set of physical exercises and that without the emotional and spiritual teaching and background the asanas are not really yoga. Yoga is believed to increase the body's stores of vital energy and to facilitate its flow through the body. Regular practice induces a deep sense of relaxation and feelings of well-being, and yoga breathing exercises counter the rapid breathing associated with the stress response if the sympathetic nervous system is triggered. It can help in depression by increasing feelings of well-being and it can counter the effects of anxiety. Yoga is particularly helpful in treating stress and insomnia.

If you are suffering from anxiety or depression, even thinking about such exercises might appear daunting. Alternatively some people rush into a new course and if they do not see immediate results give up completely. Our advice is to start gently and always tell your family doctor and ask if there are any particular problems you should be aware of that you will need to discuss with your t'ai chi or yoga teacher.

CASE HISTORY: Bob

Bob is a big strong athletic-looking man who works as a personal trainer at an exclusive private gym. His mother had died suddenly from a heart attack when he was very young. For years he had suffered from anxiety and intense panic attacks whenever he was left alone in his house, especially if his wife was away working. He had taken all manner of medication but nothing had helped him until he discovered yoga. He now practises this at least once a day and believes this has transformed his life. He is almost evangelical about its benefits for mood disorders and encourages all his clients to build yoga into their daily routines.

OTHER METHODS OF HEALING THE EMOTIONAL BRAIN

Many other methods including aromatherapy, hypnotherapy, music, meditation, massage, reiki and spiritual healing can access the emotional brain, helping to heal the mind and promote feelings of well-being. Such methods generally carry relatively few risks and can have excellent benefits in helping mood disorders. Many feed back to the emotional brain telling us that we are loved and cared for.

Chapter Eight

The Physical Toolkit

IN THIS CHAPTER WE consider the use of physical methods of treatment such as ECT, for those more seriously ill, and new methods of treatment, such as transcranial magnetic stimulation (TMS), that are just as effective as ECT but have far fewer side effects. Unfortunately the physical treatments used to treat serious depression and other mental illnesses in the past were often highly controversial, mainly because of their serious side effects. Although some are still used, they are much safer now and they are being replaced by much more effective, scientifically based methods including deep brain stimulation (DBS) which uses electrical currents to alter the workings of the brain. This is used by neurosurgeons rather than psychiatrists.

ELECTROCONVULSIVE THERAPY

Electroconvulsive therapy (ECT) is one of the most controversial treatments for serious depression.[1] It was used extensively in the 1950s and is still used today, mainly for the treatment of serious depressive illness, including for those with severe bipolar disorder. You may be offered this if all drug treatments have failed or if they have not started to take effect, especially if you are having suicidal thoughts.

Advances in ECT, including better control of the electricity used in treatment, have made the procedure much safer than in the past.[2] If you are to be treated with ECT you will first be given a short-acting barbiturate as an anaesthetic and a muscle relaxant. ECT is then administered by placing two small electrodes on the shaved scalp on one side or both sides of the head. An electric current is passed between the electrodes for a few seconds to induce convulsions, a fit or seizure. An electroencephalogram (EEG) and an electrocardiogram (ECG) are now used routinely to monitor seizure activity and heart rhythm respectively. The treatment is usually carried out for two or three days a week and lasts for several weeks.

The history of ECT

ECT dates back in the UK to late Victorian times. At that time, the medical profession, fascinated by the newly discovered force called electricity, was using it to treat all manner of conditions from psoriasis to bald patches! A medical textbook published in 1890 and written by J. McGregor-Robertson,[3] a doctor and academic from Glasgow University, reviews the then medical uses of electricity thus: 'Electricity is becoming more and more made use of in nervous afflictions connected with the brain and spinal cord and in mental illness, especially melancholia. There is a great future in store for this method of treatment. The writer has had in his own experience a few very remarkable instances where complete removal of the mental disorder followed the employment of a weak constant current of electricity to the brain. In such cases, of course, the remedy requires to be very cautiously applied.'

At the time, there was no attempt to explain scientifically how administering an electric shock to the brain could treat melancholia and no clinical trials, perhaps just the enthusiasm of doctors equipped with a new technique based on a highly fashionable new discovery.

ECT treatment was reintroduced in 1938 by the Italian neurologist Ugo Cerletti, mainly for the treatment of schizophrenia. Its use was based on the earlier work of Von Meduna,[4] who suggested a 'biological antagonism between epilepsy and schizophrenia'. Subsequent work suggested that ECT was more effective for treating depressive illness, and this continues to be its main use.

Problems and side effects

Despite advances in the procedure, problems with ECT remain:[5]

- It requires several administrations to be effective.

- It can lead to problems with memory, although it is claimed that these effects can be reduced by treating only the least dominant hemisphere.

- The relapse rate is high.

- In some cases lasting damage is caused to the patient, including tooth damage, compressional fractures to the spine, epilepsy, peripheral nerve damage and skin burns.

There are now strict guidelines for its use, including the failure of other (drug) treatments and that the patient is extremely suicidal.[6] The use of ECT under compulsion is regulated by the Mental Health Act 1983 in the UK and under similar acts elsewhere. In the US a new organisation called Psychirights,[7] has been established to oppose forced ECT. If you are concerned about being compelled to accept such treatment it is worth asking the mental health charity Mind or a similar charity for information on how to obtain legal advice.

Janet witnessed the effects on those undergoing ECT while in a mental hospital in 1982 and was on the verge of having to undergo it herself, and Jane has recorded her father's sufferings from ECT treatments in the 1950s in *Your Life in Your Hands*. She clearly remembers her mother paying out large sums of money to psychiatrists who swore by ECT. She remembers her father crying and begging not to be taken for treatment whenever it was to be administered, and she is well aware that everyone said that the treatment destroyed his personality. He was only 47 years old and was never able to work again. In his own words, 'ECT is like someone kicking a television in the hope that it might work, as opposed to calling out a television engineer who understands where the fault is and is able to repair it properly.' It is now widely acknowledged that the machines used for ECT in the 1950s – at the time Jane's father was treated – were poorly calibrated, and far too many treatments were used with often serious consequences.[8]

Nobel Prize winner Ernest Hemingway was given more than 20 ECT treatments in a mental hospital in the US.[9] He is quoted shortly afterwards as telling a friend: 'What is the sense of ruining my head and erasing my memory which is my capital and putting me out of business? It was a brilliant cure but we lost the patient.' In 1961, a few days after being released from the clinic, Hemingway committed suicide.

There are still serious concerns about the use of ECT. A survey carried out by the UK mental health charity MIND in 2006 found that 84 per cent of respondents had suffered side effects from ECT, including permanent memory loss and the inability to read, write and concentrate, as well as headaches and confusion.[10]

If you are seriously depressed and suicidal, you may be advised strongly to have ECT treatment. However, there are many anecdotes and increasingly clinical trials that show that depression and bipolar disorder can be alleviated far better by gentler methods discussed in this chapter and other chapters of the book, including using improved nutrition.[11] Unfortunately many conventional doctors and psychiatrists are unaware of them although they are highly recommended by leaders in the field such as Dr Daniel Amen and Dr David Servan-Schreiber. If all such methods of treatment have been tried and have failed we recommend that the specific problem in brain function that is causing your illness be diagnosed before ECT is used (see pages 99–101). Moreover we believe that ECT should be administered only after a doctor qualified in neurology, not a general psychiatrist, has recommended it and then only on the basis of functional brain scans that demonstrate it is essential (see pages 102–4). If you are offered ECT we strongly advise that you request transcranial magnetic stimulation treatment instead.

Vivien Leigh, the star of such classic movies as *Gone with the Wind* and *A Streetcar named Desire*, was given repeated ECT treatments to the extent it left burns on her temples.[9] Her husband, the famous actor Lawrence Olivier, was devastated by the changes in her personality and is quoted as saying: 'She is now more of a stranger to me than I could ever have imagined.' It is now thought that Vivien Leigh was in fact suffering from the side effects of medication prescribed for her tuberculosis, which can cause mental illness and psychosis.

TRANSCRANIAL MAGNETIC STIMULATION

Transcranial magnetic stimulaton (TMS) is a new non-invasive treatment that does not use drugs but uses pulses of magnetic energy to stimulate the left dorsal and frontal parts of the brain, especially the prefrontal cortex, while avoiding other areas concerned with memory. The method is being developed following the discovery that the mood of people who had MRI scans significantly improved. The magnetic pulses produce an electric field (by electromagnetic induction discovered by Faraday in 1831!) which in turn stimulates neurons in the regions of the brain to be treated. The amount of electricity generated is too small for patients to feel and the risk of a seizure is diminishingly small.

The treatment involves lying awake in a chair for about 40

minutes with two small electromagnetic coils placed in pre-selected positions on the head. The method has few if any side effects and there have been several reports in the media of people, especially in the US, who claim their lives have been transformed by TMS. Trials reported in the *British Journal of Psychiatry* showed it to be as effective as ECT in improving symptoms of depression, helping more than 40 per cent of patients but without the side effects of ECT.[12] Those treated with TMS had the same or improved cognitive and memory performance whereas there were problems especially in memory in those treated with ECT. Mark George, a clinical psychiatrist at the Medical University of South Carolina in Charleston, is quoted in a recent *New Scientist* article as saying 'In my opinion, TMS's antidepressant effects are as good as any medication we have.'[13]

Nevertheless, despite all its benefits, it should be noted that TMS is regarded as a treatment not a cure. TMS is becoming more widely available on the UK National Health Service. To be eligible for treatment in the US, patients must be between 18 and 70 years old and diagnosed with a major depressive disorder that has failed to respond to at least one antidepressant medication and not have a significant neurological disorder. It is not used on pregnant women.

PSYCHOSURGERY

This procedure is now rare but it might be recommended by your psychiatrist if you are very seriously ill with severe depression, anxiety or OCD and all other drug treatments and ECT have been tried and have failed. The procedure, formerly known as frontal lobotomy, or leucotomy in the UK, is now called NMD (neurosurgery for mental disorder). It depends on destroying the links between the unconscious mind, our older brains, and the conscious mind, our human brain, but the procedure has become more refined. The parts of the brain targeted are much smaller and are first identified using magnetic resonance imaging. Furthermore, radio frequencies rather than surgical procedures are now used.

Britain is currently one of the few countries where this sort of surgery is still permitted, and generally only on the basis that the patient gives their consent and that each case is subjected to rigorous scrutiny by appropriate ethical and clinical standards committees.

From miracle cure to medical crime against humanity

Frontal lobotomy or leucotomy was pioneered by Egas Moniz,[14] a Portuguese neurologist who in 1949 was awarded the Nobel Prize for developing and promoting the procedure. Between the mid-1930s until the early 1960s frontal lobotomy or leucotomy was heralded as a miracle cure for a wide range of mental disorders, ranging from profound depression, schizophrenia and advanced neurosyphilis to mild retardation.

The operation was carried out not only in the US but also in Japan, Britain and elsewhere, on tens of thousands of patients – an estimated 50,000 in the UK alone. The scale on which it was performed was drastically reduced in the 1970s as more and more mental disorders were treated with drugs and psychotherapy.

There are still problems in the use of NMD. Only recently we heard of someone treated using this method. The health professional recounting the case described the difficult social and economic situation that the person was in and said, without a trace of irony, it was 'enough to make anybody suicidal'. It had not occurred to her until we made the point that it would have been better to help to sort out the poor man's problems, which still remain, rather than simply use surgery to try to blunt or suppress his feelings about his situation.

The main issue is that, whether NMD is used as the treatment of choice or only as a last resort, the outcome of the procedure is unpredictable and the effects irreversible. Moreover, some patients may not be able to make an informed choice. Richard Brook, former chief executive of the mental-health charity Mind, is concerned that no leading study has properly assessed the effect of psychosurgery on an individual's personality or sought the views of those undergoing such treatment. It seems alarming that although the lobotomy is deemed one of the worst crimes in medical history, a modern form of it is still practised in Britain – and if the patient is unable to make decisions it may be performed without the patient's consent.[14] If you are seriously mentally ill, you and your supporters should consider very carefully the pros and cons of a procedure before agreeing that you be treated. Since the procedure no longer involves a surgical operation it is important to understand the difference between ECT and NMD and ensure you know which you are agreeing to (often on behalf of a loved one). If in doubt, seek advice from Mind or other such reputable charity. We believe that psychosurgery that is irreversible should be used only after all other methods of treatment have been exhausted. Proper diagnosis based on functional brain scans is essential before such a procedure is contemplated (see pages 102–4). Much better methods of changing communication between the conscious and unconscious minds based on implanting electrodes in the brain or under the skull are discussed next.

DEEP BRAIN STIMULATION (DBS)

One physical method of treating depressive illnesses, which is based on understanding the structure and physiology of the brain, involves implanting electrodes deep in specific regions of the brain. These can be stimulated repeatedly to produce remission of depressive symptoms, and it is claimed that there is a good success rate. This method, unlike NMD, has the important advantage that it is reversible – you simply turn off the current.[15]

One particularly successful method pioneered by Helen Mayberg at Emory University, Atlanta,[16] involves inserting pacemaker-like electrodes into a spot in the brain known as area 25. This she identified a decade earlier using brain scans as a key conduit of neural traffic between the 'thinking' frontal cortex and the older emotional brain. She describes the area as hyperactive 'running hot' in depressed patients – like 'a gate left open'. In early trials Mayberg and her colleagues cured 8 out of 12 severely depressed patients who had not been helped by years of drug treatments, ECT and talking therapy. Other methods, pioneered by Professor Schlaepfer, involve stimulating part of the brain's reward circuit to improve feelings of pleasure and increase motivation. The idea is to restore normal activity to faulty circuits. Preliminary results are favourable and a large clinical trial is planned.[17] Many other mood disorders, including severe anxiety conditions such as OCD, are being treated successfully using such methods.[17] There is nevertheless some risk attached to the use of these techniques, because they involve placing implants, albeit extremely thin electrodes, deep in the brain, and another approach being developed relies on inserting a patch of electrodes, about the size of a postage stamp, between the skull and the tough membrane that encases the brain. The surgery is less invasive and therefore safer than implanting DBS electrodes. The idea of cortical stimulation is to encourage neurons in the dorsolateral prefrontal cortex to develop better connections – effectively to rewire themselves. The method has previously been used to help stroke victims to improve their motor abilities and regain some independence.[17]

LIGHT THERAPY

The benefits of sunlight on mood have been known since ancient times and are apparent in the seasonal behaviour of many animals, including mammals to which we are closely related. The effects of light on our eyes and skin are transmitted to the hypothalamus which, through the pituitary gland, influences the hormonal cocktail in our bodies that can make us feel depressed and lethargic in winter and happier and livelier as spring sets in. Daylight is generally much brighter than artificial light so treatment with light in winter for SAD involves treatment with specially powerful light sources. New devices designed to simulate summer sunrise are reported to be more effective than standard exposure to light boxes. The application of light therapy should be timed according to the patient's daily rhythm of melatonin production.[18] Light therapy not only helps people affected by SAD but is also reported to help stabilise menstrual cycles, improve the quality of sleep, reduce carbohydrate cravings and enhance the response to antidepressants. Most of us benefit from being in sunlight and this is discussed further in Chapter 9.

CONCLUSIONS

Physical treatments are used mainly for serious depression when all conventional treatments have failed and the patient is considered at great risk of suicide. The latest methods of ECT and psychosurgery are much safer than older versions. Nevertheless we recommend that TMS and electrode implant methods be used to replace them. Treating depression using TMS to stimulate electrical flow in the parts of the brain that have low activity would appear to have major advantages over ECT, and implanting pacemaker-like devices in specific areas of the brain would appear to be much safer and more effective than NMD. Light therapy may help not only those suffering from SAD but other people with other types of depression.

Part Three

·

SELF-HELP AND RECOMMENDATIONS

As well as seeking help for mood disorders, it is important to learn to take better care of ourselves. Chapter 9 considers ways we can look after the emotional brain and lift the human mind and spirit, and Chapter 10 recommends measures that enhance mental well-being through improvements to the diet. By adopting helpful activities, such as eating good food and enjoying purposeful activities, and avoiding the unhelpful, like chasing wealth and being obsessed with appearance, we can go a long way towards overcoming mental illness.

Chapter 11 sets out our recommendations for a fundamental overhaul of the mental-healthcare system and, finally, we provide 12 golden guidelines to help you attain and maintain good mental health.

Chapter Nine

The Black Dog and the Human Spirit

THE BLACK DOG

WINSTON CHURCHILL famously referred to his depression as his black dog, and an excellent book of cartoons by Matthew Johnstone[1] on how to deal with depression uses a black dog as a symbol of the disease. As we have learned, depression and anxiety are both related to problems with our emotional brain, which is the part of our brain that we have in common with dogs and other mammals. Indeed, functional brain scans show that when we are depressed most of the brain's activity is in the emotional brain, with little or no activity in the human brain.

If, unlike Churchill and Johnstone, we see a black dog as a symbol not of disease but as representing our emotional brain, it can help us to understand the need to look after that part of ourselves that we so often neglect. Instead of visualising our black dog as depression we can think of it as the part of the brain that needs to be cared for if we are to improve and strengthen our mental well-being.

Janet has a lovely golden labrador called Charlie, and some of Jane's friends have two wonderful black labradors, Max and Millie. Without the overlay of the complex human mind, it is so easy to see the things that make the dogs happy. It is simple things like a good long walk, being allowed to run free and play, dig in the dirt, jump in a pond, being with others, being talked to and given attention, being cuddled or stroked, and of course being fed good food and lots of clean water.

THE HUMAN SPIRIT

According to the World Health Organisation, male suicide rates vary from less than one in 100,000 men in many Caribbean countries to levels 50 to 75 times higher in countries of the former Soviet Union, such as Ukraine, Russia and Lithuania.[2] This is not simply the result of high latitude and long winters: Iceland and Norway have much lower rates (about 19 per 100,000 males). Communist Cuba is alone among Caribbean countries in having a significant suicide rate of 24.5. In comparison, the rate in the US is 17.6.[2] It would appear that communism is not good for the human spirit. On the other hand, the Irish Republic has a male suicide rate of 18.4, almost twice that of the UK (11.8), a problem attributed by some medical specialists to the demands of the Celtic Tiger economy.[3] Although detailed analysis of the data is needed to identify causes, they nevertheless suggest that repression is not good for the human spirit but neither is rampant materialism.

BALANCING THE NEEDS OF THE BLACK DOG AND THE HUMAN MIND – YIN AND YANG

This chapter and Chapter 10 are all about looking after the black dog in all of us, as well as finding things that lift the human mind and spirit. It is important that we balance our lives and give attention to our emotional minds as well as the human mind. In terms of Chinese medicine, this is all about balancing the Yin and Yang forces.

LIFESTYLE FACTORS

In this chapter we outline ten lifestyle factors that can help to balance your life and reduce levels of stress, to help to prevent and treat anxiety and depression. The factors range from advice on how we can work on ourselves, for example, to improve our self-esteem, to the factors in our environment that we need to understand so that we can increase its positive benefits while reducing any negative impacts. They are designed to complement the ten food factors given in Chapter 10. We suggest that you start working on a few of the lifestyle factors and try to develop an achievable programme that you can take forward, rather than rushing into an ambitious and expensive plan that you cannot sustain.

Know yourself

Eliminating even small irritations and stresses from our lives can help to cut levels of circulating cortisol and hence cut our risk of switching on the amygdala and sympathetic nervous system and triggering anxiety or depression. We need to understand the things that we as individuals find particularly irritating – things that can raise our background levels of stress – and either learn how to cope with them better or eliminate them from our lives.

Senses and sensibilities

It has been suggested that people are affected by stress in different ways, according to which of their senses is affected. Thus some people become stressed by loud or ugly noises, or even noises that they feel are out of their control. Some are more disturbed by unpleasant sights, including scenes of untidiness, litter or graffiti, while others suffer if they have rough clothes or fabric next to their skin because, to them, the sense of touch is all important. Still others are badly affected by unpleasant smells. Understanding which of your senses is most likely to cause you distress can be helpful in eliminating sources of stress.

Jane knows that she falls into the first category and so she tries to avoid noisy situations. She will walk through a downpour rather than listen to a busker in a covered walkway and she avoids shopping where there is loud music. She also tricks herself into thinking she has control over noise – by listening to the radio to cut out aircraft noise, for example. On the other hand, untidiness, rough fabrics and bad smells hardly affect her at all. Janet finds that being with too many people is difficult and realises that this is because she, too, finds noise stressful. Many other people we know are very upset by ugly sights but can stand the ear bashing noise of some of the noisiest clubs and discos.

Larks and owls

It is important to work out your ideal daily pattern of activity and rest. Are you a 'lark', full of mental and physical energy as the day dawns, or an 'owl' who feels tired and lethargic in the morning and wakes up only in the afternoon and evening? Whatever your daily cycle, try to organise your life, including the type of job you do and your social life, to fit your daily rhythm.

Jane is a lark and often begins writing at 6 am, but she finds difficulty keeping awake in the evenings and prefers not to do anything demanding then. She knows that a late night is likely to make her overtired the next day because she is incapable of lying in. She does any exercise routine, usually a long walk, in the morning and prefers social breakfasts or lunches to dinners.

Janet, on the other hand, is an owl. She can't think straight in the mornings and feels she is only 'going through the motions', not really awake until at least 9 am, although she feels inspired and full of energy at midnight. Lunch is the earliest social meal she attempts.

Clearly if you have a marked daily pattern you are likely to find difficulty with shift work or intercontinental air travel. Use your analysis of your daily rhythm to cut down on stress.

There are often many other things that irritate us. Try to think what these are so you can reduce their impact.

Dear diary

Keeping a simple diary helps, because the events that trigger depressive illness can occur weeks or sometimes months before symptoms appear. Also your diary can help you to understand yourself, your daily rhythm and the things you find upsetting and stressful. Remember, too, to note the things that make you feel better and try to increase your exposure to them. Also note your positive achievements in your diary and praise yourself for them.

LIFESTYLE FACTOR 1: FOOD AND MOOD

Many of the drugs and treatments for depression appear to be based on improving energy flow in the brain. For example, increased levels of neurotransmitters in synapses help electrical charges to be transmitted between neurons, lithium helps sodium ions to cross membranes and carry electrical charges along nerve fibres, and ECT is aimed primarily at shocking the brain into allowing electricity to flow. Perhaps the effectiveness of TMS demonstrates the importance of electricity flow in the brain most clearly. It relies on principles of physics established in the early part of the nineteenth century that a changing magnetic field will cause the flow of electricity in a conductor. Jane is familiar with the technique because it has been used by geophysicists for decades to find sulphide ore deposits.

How does all this relate to our food? There is much scientific evidence that the food we eat can clog up and block the flow of energy in the brain. For example, cell membranes can become so rigid as a consequence of a bad diet that the tiny particles of sodium that carry positive electrical charges in the brain simply cannot go through them. This would explain why lithium, which is very similar to sodium chemically but is a much tinier atom, is helpful in treating bipolar disorder.

We simply may not have enough of the vitamins and amino acids in our diet, especially when we are under stress, to make the neurotransmitters that our brains need; we may lack minerals such as magnesium and lithium in the diet, which are thought to play a crucially important role in maintaining healthy brain activity. Many scientists now believe that the human brain could not have evolved without some of the foods that were available in East Africa at the time, such as seafood with its high content of lithium and iodine.[4]

Eminent scientists and doctors from Imperial College, London, the University of Pittsburgh and the National Institutes of Health in the US and elsewhere are now adamant about the role of diet in depression, including bipolar disorder, based on brain scans, epidemiological studies and clinical trials.[5]

It is important to ensure good nutrition, especially when we are under increased physical or emotional stress. It is especially important for women to maintain good nutrition during pregnancy and breast-feeding, and for everyone after a serious life-changing event such as the loss of a loved one. Try to eat good, nutritional food as described in Chapter 10, and if you are having difficulty eating have small amounts regularly to keep blood-sugar levels steady. Always drink lots of water, including as green or herbal teas, to avoid triggering a stress response because you are thirsty.

We think food is so important to mood that we have devoted a whole chapter to it (Chapter 10). We hope you will find this a comprehensive and practical account of the dietary factors implicated in anxiety and depression and be able to make the simple changes suggested to help prevent and treat your illness.

LIFESTYLE FACTOR 2: MAY THE FORCE BE WITH YOU

There is no doubt that, whatever the illness, having a faith helps, and all the scientific evidence supports this.[6] The acceptance of a higher being is fundamental to the work of Alcoholics Anonymous, and yoga is not considered to be yoga without its spiritual aspects. Moreover, the latest scientific evidence shows that humans, as a species, are unique in having a part of the brain capable of having religious experiences and all the evidence shows that even Buddhist chanting or saying the rosary helps to give us peace of mind. Why, then, have so many people lost their faith in God and replaced it with an empty materialistic and celebrity culture?

First, we need to return to the simple concept that God is good. We all know what goodness is, and although God may be beyond human comprehension we can all recognise the forces of goodness and those of (the d)evil. Most stories that we enjoy from childhood onwards, whether *The Lord of the Rings* or a Harry Potter book, are about the triumph of good over evil. In *Star Wars*, those battling on the side of goodness are repeatedly given the simple blessing 'May the force be with you'. In fact the film is based on the Taoist religion of ancient China, which introduced concepts such as Yin and Yang, which are still the basis of Chinese medicine. The Tao is a force that pervades the universe, is the essence of individuals and is the way to lead your life; sometimes the word Tao is translated as 'the way' or 'the path'. Taoism is all about living in tune with nature rather than manipulating the environment.

There are several reasons why so many people have lost their faith. First, religion appears to be behind so many human conflicts. Fundamentalists within Islam, Christianity and Judaism are presently fuelling conflict and terror throughout the world. There are even problems between different groups within the Christian religion. Difficulties between Catholics and Protestants led to incredible evil in Northern Ireland until the beginning of the twenty-first century. Religion as sometimes practised is often simply a form of human tribalism that has forgotten that, quite simply, God is good. Wearing particular clothes or eating only certain types of food are cultural and often stem from public-health measures introduced in the past by tribal leaders. For example, avoiding pork probably arose because it used to carry tapeworms. Accumulating vast riches, issuing orders to kill others, subjugating women or teaching that the use of condoms is a mortal sin, even in parts of the world where AIDS is endemic, are mainly actions to enhance the standing of power-hungry old men. None are in the teachings of the great prophets or religious leaders such as the Buddha, Jesus Christ or Mohammed. They have nothing to do with a God of goodness.

Another reason is that some so-called intellectuals write books and make TV programmes telling us that there is no God. We are even told that God is a delusion and that religion involves 'juvenile superstitions'. These people are usually Darwinist biologists. First let us say that we agree entirely with Darwin's scientific findings (Jane is, after all, an Earth scientist) but we cannot see any conflict with the book of Genesis. Indeed the latest scientific findings show that all modern humans are descended from a common ancestor, known to biological anthropologists as African Eve.[7] The problem seems to be in the too literal understanding of Genesis, which is metaphorical. Missing the metaphor has often caused problems in literature. For example, D. H. Lawrence's wonderful book *Lady Chatterley's Lover* was an attack on sterile materialism in the person of Sir Clifford Chatterley in contrast with the happiness and satisfaction of nature in the person of Mellors the gamekeeper, but it was almost totally misunderstood by people ignorant of the style of metaphorical writing that was popular in the early part of the twentieth century.

The main problem with biologists against God, however, is that they do not know what they do not know, and their central assumption that they have minds that can appreciate and understand everything. One wise old professor once explained to Jane how the brightest students often came out of examinations thinking they had done badly because they realised how vast the subject was and how little their answer contributed, whereas those with more limited minds frequently overestimated how well they had done.

Darwinian biology is really not too difficult for most of us to understand. On the other hand all the really brilliant physical scientists that we know, such as physicists, chemists and mathematicians who deal with difficult-to-understand abstract concepts, including the origin of the universe, believe that there must be a God. Jane clearly recalls sitting next to a distinguished physicist at a dinner in Yale who explained to her the mathematical evidence that there are at least 11 dimensions in the universe but that we as human beings can appreciate only four – a three-dimensional object moving through space and time. The biologists against God seem to assume that their minds are capable of appreciating anything and everything. They should perhaps bear in mind that a fly or a worm cannot appreciate what a human being is, even when we are actually touching them. How, then, can these biologists know that they have a brain capable of appreciating what God is? They can't. They are just supremely arrogant!

A recent article in *New Scientist* entitled 'God's place in a rational world' pointed out that faith, religion, culture and emotion are all part of the human condition and that religious beliefs help us to deal with the unpredictability and unknown nature of our environment. They appear to have evolved in a similar way to our ability to stand upright and are as much a part of our humanity.[8]

We encourage you to believe in a higher being, quite simply a force for goodness, and to pray for help and comfort. Try to do this in a quiet way, and if someone finds a different way that they find helpful let them be. You might find joining a religious group helpful, but be careful to avoid extremists, fundamentalists and cults which have little to do with the force of goodness. Also try to avoid religions that rant on about mortal sin. This is unhelpful and counterproductive in most situations and is simply aimed at control.

If we do something bad, it affects our health and in some cases our own guilt can make us seriously ill. Shakespeare's Lady Macbeth and Raskolnikov, the central character in Dostoevsky's brilliant novel *Crime and Punishment,* are examples from literature of a person's guilt eating away at their minds. It has been pointed out that there are some aspects of guilt that are neither rational nor moral.[9] We all know that we cannot undo the past but we can learn to do better in the future. At a very simple level we need to feel sorrow and regret for what we have done wrong, whatever that is, and believe that if we truly repent we can be forgiven and resolve, with support, not to repeat our wrongdoing. The best religions give us simple rules to live by, such as the Ten Commandments, and help and support to follow them. They also help us to find forgiveness and a way forward.

LIFESTYLE FACTOR 3: SELF-ESTEEM – THE INS AND OUTS

This is a complex issue in which it is important to find the right balance between personality and appearance. Society's present obsession with celebrity culture and the emphasis on presentation rather than substance is causing distress to many people, especially the young. Improve your self-esteem by working on your appearance, but don't take this to extremes.

It is important to work on people skills such as conversation – and listening, too. It is easy to improve these skills with a little honest self-examination. If you know you always talk too much, learn to listen more and you will find people respond better to you. On the other hand, if you never have anything to say try listening to some good radio programmes such as Radio 4 or the World Service of the BBC or start reading a good newspaper to improve your knowledge and confidence. Most people tend to like being with people with sympathetic personalities who are interested in other people and issues other than themselves. This can be particularly difficult if you are anxious or depressed. Jane clearly remembers emptying part of a room of people when she explained she was ill with anxiety at a friend's birthday party. One woman stayed to talk to her, however; she reassured Jane that she was not being boring and they are still firm friends. Try to work on things that build your self-esteem gradually and seek out friends who are not only understanding and supportive but who value you.

Trophy people

Unfortunately, people's lives can be made miserable by comparing themselves (and sometimes their partner!) with the images of tall thin young women and muscular lean men promoted by the media. This can be a particular problem for those with low self-esteem. People who set great store by material possessions can be strongly influenced by physical appearance and may choose a 'trophy' partner who provides little of the type of companionship that is the basis of a good long-term relationship. One rich dentist who became badly depressed because his relationships with women were always 'a disaster' was asked to think what type of person his red Porsche car would attract. All his behaviour was aimed at finding a partner who showed off his status rather than finding someone whose company he enjoyed. Another man, who has had similar problems, said without hesitation when asked what sort of women he found attractive, 'blondes', while another replied that he liked 'very slim brunettes' – with no mention of the sort of person they enjoy spending time with. Women, of course, can be just as superficial. Some highly intelligent men can have low self-esteem because they compare themselves (and feel women do too) with good-looking pop stars and footballers, however boring and inarticulate they are.

Real people and plastic people

Classic novels like *Jane Eyre*, *Middlemarch* and *Pride and Prejudice* were about personality first and physical appearance last as the basis for attraction but, sadly, these books no longer have the influence they once did. The type of physical 'perfection' first promoted by Hollywood seems to have taken over. Such physical 'perfection' is often achieved with plastic surgery, cosmetic dentistry, wigs and hair extensions, and photographs that are frequently 'enhanced' using a computer. Sometimes people have had so much cosmetic work done on their face that talking to them can be like talking to a mask – and often, inside, they are still unhappy.

Many celebrities, especially models, are what our grandmothers would have described as painfully thin or even scrawny, and the press is full of stories of young women starving themselves to death as anorexia or bulimia takes over their lives. Many anorexics we know have smoked and taken drugs to suppress their appetite and have developed crippling osteoporosis as well as anxiety and depression because of a lack of proper nutrition. We all become highly stressed when we are hungry, and deficiencies in minerals and vitamins can also cause mental illness. The subject of eating disorders is complex; there are no simple answers and each case is unique. Nevertheless, the overall message is clear: try to ignore plastic images of how people 'should' look!

Ageing

There is huge pressure in today's society, to look, sound and behave in a youthful way. We are constantly bombarded with advertisements on how to keep our hair, skin and overall appearance looking young, with images in the media again often based on plastic surgery and fake images produced with the help of the computer. Depression associated with a loss of youthful good looks tends to hit those who have relied mainly on their physical attractiveness as the foundation of their personality and social attributes. Try to develop other aspects of your personality and abilities, as well as looking well-groomed in a style appropriate for your age.

Making the most of yourself

Studies show that if you look better your self-esteem will improve[10] – but try to be realistic. Try to think of someone who is your type, who you admire, who looks good – and try to learn from them. The first thing to do if you are overweight or have poor skin or hair is to have good nutritious food. Follow the simple recommendations for healthy eating in the Plant Programme (Chapter 10). This won't make you very thin, but it will help you reach the weight that is right for you and it won't cause you to become stressed in the way that many slimming diets do if they are based on very restricted calorie intake. Your skin, hair and nails should also improve. If you can't shed the weight by following the Plant Programme, ask your doctor to have your thyroid checked to make sure it is not underactive, because this can lead to weight gain and depression. Also try doing some exercise. This helps your appearance and it is one of the best ways of improving mood (see pages 189–90).

If you can afford to do so, go to a good hairdresser and have your hair restyled. Some people's whole appearance can be lifted by a new hairdo. Try on wigs beforehand or look at an image-processor picture with the suggested new look to ensure that you will like the result and not be made to feel even more miserable. Many hairdressers give concessions for elderly people and sometimes you can get a cheaper hairdo if it is done by a student trainee.

A recent Japanese study showed how much make-up can help women's self-esteem.[11] You could employ a lifestyle coach or colour adviser to work out the best look for you, but if that is too expensive simply go to a department store and ask one of the people selling cosmetics to make up your face. Try to interact with them to develop the most flattering look that you feel comfortable with. If the products are too expensive just try to remember the types of products and shades that were used. Ideally buy a set and then match them with a less expensive range. Try to avoid perfume and fragrances. These often contain chemicals such as artificial musks and preservatives, which accumulate in the body.

Wearing clothes that make you look good helps a lot, but try not to become a 'fashion victim' because this can waste money and time and cause stress. Most women's and men's magazines have articles to help choose the clothes most flattering for different heights and builds. Colour consultants advise on the most flattering colours – or you can find simple guidelines on the Internet to identify whether you are a spring, summer, autumn or winter type.

Clothes and physical stress

Try to wear clothes and shoes that you feel comfortable in and that keep you at the right temperature. Remember that wearing clothes or shoes that are too tight or hurt or that make you too hot or too cold can pile on the stress. Wear layers of clothing that can be adjusted according to the temperature. In winter, you might find it helpful to wear thermal underwear which is now difficult to distinguish from normal underwear. In hot countries, try and find natural shade or cool down in old stone or brick buildings during the day. Sleep with good natural ventilation, with mosquito nets as necessary at night.

Properly dressed?

Above all, try to smile at people. This will improve their reaction to you and help lift your mood. One lovely elderly lady we know said she was always told as a child that she was not properly dressed until she had put a smile on her face. Now in her late seventies, she is still very popular with young and old alike. According to Dr Servan-Schreiber a real smile that involves the eyes as well as the mouth is a simple physiological marker of harmony between our cognitive human brain and our emotional brain. It tells us that the person is in a state of harmony with what they think in their cognitive brain and what they feel in their emotional brain. It is also the simplest way of feeding back the message to inner self that all is well.

LIFESTYLE FACTOR 4: THE NIGHTMARE OF THE AMERICAN DREAM

Recently there was a quotation in a magazine from Princess Beatrice, the eldest daughter of the Duke and Duchess of York, on a family holiday that took in a poor part of India. 'Isn't it strange,' she said, 'that people who have nothing are so happy, when other people who have so much often aren't happy at all?' Unfortunately, material things, above a basic level, rarely bring happiness. One wealthy Danish man that Jane used to know, who appeared to have everything that money could buy, from expensive homes to yachts, but who had never found time for relationships, simply threw himself off his balcony one day. His suicide note made it clear how sterile and unsatisfying he thought his life had become.

Many people who succumb to depression are high achievers, still driven by their childhood experiences to show how successful they are. They put too much effort into achieving success and flaunting symbols of success and far too little time into themselves and their relationships. Such people can also cause themselves much stress by envying and trying to compete with others. The famous play *American Buffalo* by David Mamet was an attack on the American Dream and the need to have the latest car, refrigerator or other consumable destined to turn into junk. The play demonstrates that in the end if we pursue this lifestyle all that is left is junk – and dysfunctional, unhappy people. Unfortunately, the American Dream is continuing on its destructive path across the globe. In Britain, many of our cities are becoming ringed by huge gleaming storage units, first seen in suburban America, where people can store all of the spare 'stuff' they have accumulated! Perhaps one of the most ridiculous symbols of status is the car. The idea that we judge each other by the metal box we repackage ourselves in is one idea we can reject and not be pressured by. Next time someone tries to impress you with their latest 'tin', just smile to yourself and remember the ridiculous Toady in Kenneth Grahame's wonderful book, *The Wind in the Willows*.

Family and friendships should be based on support and mutual trust, not destructive negative competition, rivalry and envy. The importance of good relationships is also stressed by Dr Servan-

Schreiber. In commenting on how to reverse the trend of dramatically increasing prescriptions of antidepressants, he states: 'If someone asked me where to begin to reverse this trend, I would reply that we need to start by confronting the violence in daily relationships, in couples, with our children, or our neighbours, and in the workplace. We need to become more respectful of the needs of our emotional brain for harmony and connectedness. There is no way around what evolution has wired us to want and feel in relationships.'[12]

Money worries

This is too complex an issue to do justice to here, but one of the important consequences of trying to fulfil the American Dream is spending too much money and in some cases becoming compulsive shoppers, simply buying too many things.

We suggest that if you have money problems you contact your local Citizens' Advice Bureau. Their help is free and, if necessary, they can refer you to local professionals such as accountants, financial advisors, lawyers and debt advisors whom you can trust. Never turn to a 'loan shark' or anyone else with a vested interest in lending you money at greatly inflated interest rates.

LIFESTYLE FACTOR 5: TIME WELL SPENT

One of the most unpleasant symptoms of anxiety and depression is that time appears to pass incredibly slowly. It feels like the five minutes that never end when we have arrived early and are waiting for a shop to open. On the other hand, if we are interested or absorbed in something time appears to pass incredibly quickly. We often remark 'doesn't time fly!' when we have been chatting happily with our friends. This is because the brain uses two completely different methods of time keeping, and unfortunately when we are ill with anxiety or depression it uses the 'will this never end' system. It is helpful to most people with anxiety or depression to try to find something to occupy their time and their mind.

Lewis Wolpert's book *Malignant Sadness: the Anatomy of Depres-*

sion[13] concludes by repeating the advice given at the end of Burton's classic book *The Anatomy of Melancholy*,[14] 'Be not idle'. This is excellent advice. Churchill famously kept working, writing books, painting and even building brick walls to deal with his 'black dog'. Just think what he achieved.

Work

It is now generally recognised that in most situations work is a powerful aid to recovery from anxiety and depression, and it is vital that people keep their jobs or are helped back into work if this is possible.[15] If you are in work but concerned that your mental state is affecting your performance, enlist the help and support of the human resources or personnel department at your place of work; they should regard anxiety and depression as a temporary illness or, in the case of chronic illness, a disability.

However, sometimes it is the type of work or the job you do that is the main source of stress. If that is the case, think carefully about beneficial changes you can make. If they are minor, try to make them with the support of those you work with. If they involve a major career change, consider and discuss this fully when you are feeling well before doing anything irretrievable. Ideally take leave, unpaid if necessary, to try out your new role before committing to it.

If you are out of work and would like to find a job, try working for charity until something else comes along. This will look much better on your CV than saying you simply stayed at home. Many towns have local drop-in centres where you can volunteer.[16]

Entertainment, interests and hobbies

The way you spend your spare time can also affect your mental wellbeing. For most people social activities help most but any absorbing activity can be beneficial. If you are vulnerable to anxiety or depression it is best to avoid watching the violent 'in-your-face' movies, television programmes or computer games that are around today because they leave nothing to the imagination and can really pile on the stress. Research carried out in Indianapolis University in the US showed that the brains of people playing violent video games showed less activity in the higher centres of the brain, which are concerned with concentration and self-control, and more activity in the amygdala, indicating a high degree of emotional arousal.[17] Watching a car chase or violent scene can increase heart rate and breathing, reflecting the release of stress hormones. Try to determine if this applies to you; if it does, try to avoid such 'entertainment'. It does not mean you are a wimp: you just don't like violence and that's fine.

Try to cut down generally on the amount of time you spend looking at your television or computer screen. Working on computers can be very isolating and often leads to loneliness. If possible, talk to people in person or over the phone rather than e-mailing or texting them. Try to limit the amount of time you spend talking on a mobile phone. Scientists have known for some time that, although weak, microwaves can cause changes to the blood–brain barrier, potentially causing the brain's defences against toxins and infection to be weakened.[18]

Find good ways to unwind that make you feel better over the long term. Choose books, movies, TV programmes, etc., that enhance your mood. Consider reading books with friends and then discussing them together. This can help greatly to improve your knowledge, confidence and self-esteem – but remember that everyone else is entitled to their own opinion! It is not a matter of winning the approval of others, it is just learning to contribute your thoughts. Eventually, as your confidence develops, you might wish to consider joining a book club. Going round an art exhibition, listening to a concert, eating out with friends or family, enjoying good conversation, or seeing a good play or a film are all good ways to relax and take your mind off your problems.

Dancing is fun, sociable and involves exercise and music. Joining in with some sporting activities can also be helpful. On the other hand, watching some sports can really pile on the stress, so ensure that you can cope. Playing card games, dominoes or darts can help, but once again do not become involved in stressful situations. Some bridge players can be lethal!

Many people suffering from depression have little interest in anything. They are entirely inwardly focused and to them time seems to pass very slowly. Again, these symptoms cannot be reversed suddenly and dramatically but, over time, taking up an interest or hobby can help greatly. We know of people who have suffered from anxiety or depression for years and whose lives have been transformed by their developing an interest in an allotment, by learning gardening skills or by learning to ring bells at their local church. Try to think of the things you might have an interest in and move into them gradually, ideally with the support of a partner or a friend who will work with you. Make sure that the hobby does not turn into a competition, though: it should be purely something that gives you pleasure and it really does not matter if your cabbages are better than the Joneses'!

LIFESTYLE FACTOR 6: EXERCISE

There is mounting evidence that physical exercise can greatly improve the symptoms of depression and that it is particularly beneficial in reducing anxiety. According to *The Desktop Guide to Complementary and Alternative Medicine: an evidence-based approach*, 'the indications are that both aerobic and non-aerobic forms of exercise are effective'.[19] There is also evidence from clinical trials that aerobic exercise such as walking, cycling and swimming is as effective as psychological or pharmaceutical treatment. New evidence from brain scans shows that exercise not only increases muscle power but also helps grow new brain cells.[20] This is particularly important if cells have been lost as a result of stress.

If you are suffering from a depressive illness, even thinking about such exercises might appear daunting. Alternatively, some people rush into a new course and if they do not see immediate results give up completely. Our advice is to start gently. There is no better exercise than a walk in daylight. Start off with a short walk and work up gradually, remembering to praise yourself for any progress. Use a pedometer to work up to at least 10,000 steps a day. Other simple changes you can make include doing shopping on foot or bicycle and walking rather than driving your children to school. Using the car as little as possible will reduce your stress levels and improve your physical and mental well-being. As your health improves, consider adding something more challenging like t'ai chi or yoga to your regime (see pages 157–9).

LIFESTYLE FACTOR 7: REST AND RELAXATION

Scientific evidence strongly suggests that relaxation can have profoundly positive effects on the physical, psychological and spiritual well-being of individuals and that 'doing nothing' should be seen as an important part of staying healthy, not as laziness.[21] There are many excellent methods available including massage, hypnosis, meditation and breathing exercises to help you to slow down. Many have been shown clinically to help mental well-being. Massage, for example, has been shown to reduce symptoms of anxiety, depression and insomnia, as well as reducing cortisol levels.[22]

Although doing nothing is good relaxation for some people, there are others, particularly those suffering from anxiety, for whom doing nothing simply provides an opportunity for the mind to go racing off on all its usual repetitive worries and woes. For such people, doing nothing (such as lying in the sun) is no relaxation at all. What they need is something to occupy the mind, presenting just the right level of challenge: not too much, not too little. Examples might be crossword puzzles, sudoku, cooking or gardening.

Some people may live in very stressful situations, for example on crime-ridden and drug-ridden estates. It is particularly important that such people find some respite. Ideally they should try to go out for walks in safe places or spend time with people they find caring and supportive.

The important thing, especially if you are feeling anxious or depressed, is to find some way of relaxing. It does not have to be anything in particular, as long as it is something you enjoy. It might be listening to music, wandering around antique shops or reading a magazine. The important thing is to take time out for a few hours a week with no prescheduled activities, 'shoulds' or 'musts'. Also, try to have at least one full day a week for rest and relaxation.

Sleep is particularly important in maintaining and restoring our mental health. Light pollution and noise can cause particular problems. If you live in an area where there are bright street lights that are kept on all night, use heavy curtains or wear the sort of eye masks supplied by airlines to provide the degree of darkness that promotes sleep. In the case of noise, try to discuss and resolve problems amicably with neighbours and only take matters to the authorities if absolutely necessary. Wear earplugs, or listen to your radio or music in the background to cut out traffic or aircraft noise.

Good tips for getting to sleep include establishing a routine, almost a ritual, that includes a relaxing warm bath with lavender oil and Epsom salts, eating a bowl of porridge before going to bed and listening to relaxation tapes. If you buy a tape to send you to sleep, make sure it does not at some point command you to 'be wide awake'. Unfortunately many do! Try to avoid stressful activities before going to bed and avoid heavy meals based on animal protein after lunchtime.

LIFESTYLE FACTOR 8: TRAVEL

One eminent psychotherapist we know always reminds people that it is not possible to run away from the mind however far they travel. Unfortunately, many people now take holidays that are a sort of status symbol and involve them in flying long distances to reach exotic destinations. Intercontinental flight across time zones can cause stress to the body by disturbing its internal daily rhythms, especially if there are also sudden changes in temperature, which the body has no time to adapt to. Sometimes the stress shows up as depressive illness a few weeks later, when it may be wrongly attributed to the come-down after the holiday. If intercontinental flights affect you badly, think carefully before travelling across time zones – it may suit you better simply to fly north or south.

If you suffer from SAD in winter months and you can afford to do so, take holidays in the sun at this time. (Otherwise try to obtain light therapy using a light box which you can use at home or at the office. They are available under the NHS and other national health-care systems.)

Driving is another stressful way of travelling. Study after study has shown that driving increases circulating levels of stress hormones and the excretion of neurotransmitters in urine.[23] Several factors are thought to contribute, including the personality of the driver, their aggression and life circumstances, and particular situations such as being on a tight schedule or driving in congested or other unpleasant conditions. Try to use public transport whenever you can. This is much better for you and for the environment.

Try to visualise what would be your ideal holiday, a holiday that would make you feel better. A walk along a beautiful beach, visiting historic buildings, being surrounded by trees and gardens, or mountains and lakes, or simply going on a shopping trip. Then work out the nearest place that fulfils your dream and plan to go there with the minimum of air travel or driving. Consider going by train and boat and hiring a car, or better still a bicycle, when you arrive.

LIFESTYLE FACTOR 9: YOUR ENVIRONMENT

Towns and cities

One important clue to the causes of the increase in the rates of anxiety and depression is that the increase has been in parallel with other diseases such as obesity. In their book *Urban Sprawl and Public Health*, Frumkin, Frank and Jackson describe disease 'syndemics' (epidemics of different diseases affecting similar groups of people) in the US today.[23] They suggest that such syndemics are brought about by problems with the built environment, particularly the interrelated problems of suburban sprawl and inner-city decline. Jackson, who is the State Public Health Officer for California, attributes the syndemic of obesity, diabetes, heart disease, osteoporosis, stress and depression in the suburbs there to the lack of physical exercise and social interaction because of the poor design of the built environment and the overwhelming influence of the car.

People in inner city areas, 'those left behind without automobiles', on the other hand are said to be affected by the syndemic of cardiovascular disease, cirrhosis, homicide, cancers, serious mental illness and HIV/AIDS – reflecting poverty, unemployment, drug and alcohol abuse, domestic and gang violence, and unsafe sex.

Importantly, studies of mental illness in relation to the urban environment clearly show that it increases as population density increases, even after all other factors have been discounted.[24]

The problem of depression in America's suburbs has also been described by James Howard Kunstler as follows: 'Most Americans live in suburban habitats that are isolating, disaggregated and neurologically punishing. Placed in such an environment, even a theoretically healthy individual would sooner or later succumb to the kind of despair and anomie that we have labelled "depression". The emotional toll of the American Dream is steep. What we see all over our nation is a situational loneliness of the most extreme kind ...

'The pervasive situational loneliness of being stuck alone in your car, alone in your work cubicle, alone in your apartment, alone at the supermarket, alone at the video rental shop – because that's how American daily life has come to be organised – is the injury to which the insult of living in degrading, ugly, frightening and monotonous surroundings is added. Is it any wonder that Americans resort to the few things available that afford even a semblance of contentment: eating easily obtainable and cheap junk food and popping a daily dose of Paxil or Prozac to stave off feelings of despair that might actually be a predictable response to settings and circumstances of our lives?'[25]

Concern about the impact of the built environment on public health has been expressed by the US Department of Health and Human Services, who indicate a need for better public health policy to improve the health and quality of life of all Americans.[26]

A similar pattern can be recognised in the UK. Despite armies of social 'scientists', planners and architects, much of what we have built in recent years are estates of identical little boxes with their garages and hard standing for cars, consuming ever more of the green space that we can ill afford to lose. Often such estates are designed as commuter housing but without any public transport, cycle tracks or safe attractive paths, and they lack any centres that would encourage social interaction. Many are also 'food deserts' where it is difficult to buy fresh fruit or vegetables.

We have systematically destroyed well-built Victorian cottages and terraced housing, with the communities that had grown up around them, and replaced them with soulless third-rate multi-storey concrete blocks without gardens or spaces for the young to play safely. All this under the influence of trendy architects and unthinking planners, who usually live in attractive Regency or Victorian terraces. There is the occasional architect-built 'statement building', usually aimed at other architects or winning prizes, which always and predictably fails to fit in with its surroundings. In Cambridge the Lyon Court building built by Queens' College in 1989 wrecks the famous view of 'the backs'. In Oxford, Bill Bryson imagines a committee of finely educated minds in Merton College saying to themselves 'we've been putting up handsome buildings since 1264; let's have an ugly one for a change', a point of view to which the planning authorities concur, with 'Why not? Plenty worse in Basildon.'[27]

Since the 1950s little or nothing has been built in the UK that would help to rebuild communities or provide a sense of place and belonging. The towns of Reading, Basingstoke and Swindon are just three examples of town centres that now comprise jumbles of ugly buildings in clashing styles, lacking any sense of place. The Office of the Deputy Prime Minister, headed by John Prescott, led a campaign to develop yet more houses in the already stressed environment of south-east England – a movement widely referred to as 'Prescott's dash for trash'. Unfortunately this is now being championed by Gordon Brown.

In America, the central problem is now regarded as development for cars rather than people. To quote Frumkin, Frank and Jackson again: 'Dependence on the automobile has contributed to air pollution, threatening respiratory health and increasing the risk of injuries among drivers, passengers and pedestrians. With less walking and bicycling, sedentary lifestyles contribute to the epidemics of obesity, diabetes and heart disease. The effects of suburban sprawl on mental health and social capital may be profound. We routinely find ourselves in environments that are dispiriting and ugly – miles of strip malls, vast parking lots, neighbourhoods with no way to walk and with no places to which to walk.'[28]

The voices that have spoken out against this type of development in the UK, most notably Prince Charles, have been derided. The type of traditional housing that, in the past, created strong communities in Britain and offered some humanity have been dismissed as 'pastiches'.

'Smart growth'

Fortunately, the tide is now turning. In the UK, many local and regional authorities have accepted the benefits of green space that encourages people to walk, run, cycle and play and to meet and talk to each other in safe attractive surroundings, and are working to develop more. The best schemes involve interaction with local communities. Some of the most enlightened authorities are stripping out the urban motorways that sliced through their communities and are replacing them with attractive pedestrianised recreational areas with park-and-ride schemes to keep cars out of city centres. According to Frumkin, Frank and Jackson: 'We are now rediscovering some old wisdom and identifying principles for healthy place making in the new century. At its best, smart growth is like a medicine that treats a multitude of diseases (including depression). In the medical world such an intervention would be regarded as miraculous.'[28]

Nevertheless, especially in the US and UK, we still have a legacy of built environments that are totally unsuitable for human communities. We must be careful not to repeat this mistake in the future just because some politician is trying to win popular votes in the short term.

Humans and green space

In 1984 a paper described how patients in a surgical ward in a hospital in Italy who had had operations to remove their gall bladders and whose beds were on one side of the ward were routinely discharged more than three days earlier than patients on the other side of the ward.[29] There was no statistical difference in the age of the patients, the seriousness of their conditions or any other simple physical variable that could account for this. It was eventually realised that the patients discharged early were from the side of the ward that looked out onto trees and natural light, while patients on the side of the ward with only pictures lit by artificial lighting fared less well. Such research is now influencing modern hospital design, and it is also underlining the importance of green space for physical and mental well-being generally.

A recent article in *The Times* suggested that ecotherapies for depression such as country walks and care farms, where patients are prescribed agricultural work, are being ignored as Britain becomes ever more reliant on chemical drug treatments. The mental-health charity Mind is quoted as saying that ecotherapy has the potential to help millions of people and would be vastly cheaper than antidepressant drugs. Mind also pointed out that the Netherlands had 600 care farms operating as part of the health service, while Britain had only 43, and none was dedicated to mental health.[30]

The direct mental-health benefits of access to green space include[31]:

- Improved self-awareness, self-esteem and mood.

- Reduction of negative feelings such as anger, anxiety, fear and frustration.

- Improved ability to recover from stressful episodes.

- Alleviation of the symptoms of anxiety and depression, including insomnia, tension, irritability, headaches and indigestion.

- Improved psychological health, especially emotional and cognitive function.

- Restored capacity for attention and concentration.

Interestingly, living in low-density housing in the suburbs is not helpful: 'suburban neurosis' is variously attributed to factors such as social isolation or the need to commute long distances.[32]

Ideally, we should all try to spend time out of doors in a park or communal garden each day.[33] Unfortunately, green space in some urban areas may not be safe, but even if you live in an unsafe area there are things you can do such as walking down tree-lined streets or going to a garden centre. If you live in a city you can always catch a bus to visit a nearby park or nearby countryside. Britain generally has many wonderful urban parks and fabulous countryside. Try to spend as much time there as you can.

If you are housebound, try to look out of a window at trees, birds and sky. Encourage wild birds by feeding them. If all else fails, try to have some plants to look at; even a few in a window box or on a balcony can help. Growing creeping plants can improve some of the bleakest buildings.

We all need to make it clear to our politicians and civil servants that we wish to live in sustainable communities designed for humans, not humans in cars. We also need to make it clear that we cannot afford to give up any more of our green space to housing and urban development. If we do, many more people are likely, quite literally, to lose their minds!

LIFESTYLE FACTOR 10: AVOIDING SUBSTANCES HARMFUL TO OUR NERVOUS SYSTEM

There are many chemicals, ranging from recreational drugs and alcohol to man-made industrial chemicals and pesticides, that can damage our nervous system and contribute to anxiety and depression. Here we tell you about some of the most important ones and give you advice on cutting down your exposure to them.

Drugs and self-medication

Never be persuaded to experiment with recreational drugs, including tobacco, or abuse alcohol. You would be playing with fire and could become an addict. If you feel you already have a problem with drugs, including tobacco or alcohol, seek help. Ask your GP to refer you to your nearest drug and alcohol team. Alcoholics Anonymous and Narcotics Anonymous are wonderful, international organisations that have regular meetings to help people deal with their problems. The NHS in the UK offers support in quitting tobacco smoking.

Some people endlessly pop over-the-counter, non-prescription pills. Some of these can be harmful. For example, many antacids contain aluminium in a potentially bioavailable form which can cause neurotoxicity. Try to deal with the fundamental problem with the help of your doctor. Jane's book *Eating for Better Health* will help you deal with many irritating health problems.

Chemicals in the environment

According to recent studies, hundreds of industrial chemicals that are toxic to the human brain are produced in large quantities (more than one million tonnes a year), and many are likely to be present in our environment, food and consumer goods.[34]

Many of the chemicals of concern are highly fat-soluble, so they can become concentrated in the brain, which is 60 per cent fat, and in the fatty myelin sheaths of the nervous system. Moreover, the blood–brain barrier, which normally protects us from such chemicals, is leakier when we are under stress, abuse alcohol or are affected by other chemicals. Many neurotoxic chemicals are highly persistent, and recent surveys by the WWF have shown that there are elevated levels of a cocktail of potentially toxic chemicals in most people's blood.[35]

In June 2007 the European Union introduced legislation to control the use of hazardous chemicals, so things are likely to improve in Europe, but most of the rest of the world, including North America, is lagging behind. Remember that there are three main ways that chemicals can enter the body: by breathing them in as fumes, dusts and particulates; by taking them in with food and drink, including from unwashed hands; and by absorption through the skin or as a result of injection.

Heavy metals

There is evidence that our bodies now contain far more heavy metals (such as mercury, lead and cadmium) than those of our ancestors, and it has been suggested that this is an important factor in the rise of depressive illness. Some heavy metals are well known to be neuro-toxic and are associated with severe mental illness.[36] Exposure to cadmium or methyl mercury have been shown in laboratory animals to produce significant decreases in brain-stem serotonin levels, for example, while exposure to lead also decreases brain-stem noradrenaline activity.[37]

Some of the most distressing symptoms of mercury poisoning (extreme excitability and nervous agitation) are because it interferes with the cycle of the excitory neurotransmitter glutamate. It is nicknamed 'the mad-hatter syndrome' after the famous character in Lewis Carroll's classic book, *Alice in Wonderland*, because hatters in Victorian England used mercury to preserve the fabrics they used to make hats.

Mercury continues to be used for dental fillings and as a preservative in many vaccines, including influenza vaccines and the measles, mumps and rubella (MMR) vaccine. Indeed, some scientists attribute autism in small children to the mercury preservative thiomersal, which is about 20 times as toxic as mercury itself and was used in the MMR vaccine until recently.[38] So ensure you accept only thiomersal-free vaccinations and injections. In general, if you have mercury fillings you may be advised to leave them but we recommend against new ones.

In addition to increased exposure from such sources, the background level of mercury globally has increased since the 1980s, especially as a result of the burning of fossil fuels to generate energy in China and India. Considerable quantities of mercury are accumulating in fish in the oceans, to the extent that the American Food and Drug Administration and the UK Food Standards Agency have issued warnings to pregnant and nursing mothers not to consume more than the equivalent of one small can of tuna or other ocean fish a week.[39] In Chapter 10 we give advice on good sources of sea foods that are likely to contain lesser amounts of mercury than ocean fish.

Lead is also widely acknowledged to be a serious neurotoxin. Until recently, it was used in domestic plumbing and paints and as an anti-knock agent in petrol. Many historians and archaeologists attribute the bizarre behaviour of the Romans during the decline of the Roman Empire to lead poisoning. The Romans used lead not only for plumbing and storage vessels, but because they liked the sweet taste of its salts they added them to their wine and puddings! One of the toxic effects of lead is that it interferes with serotonin production. In one study, monkeys exposed to lead experimentally became so dangerously aggressive that the study had to be halted.[40]

Exposure to lead has been reduced dramatically following legislation in the 1970s to remove it from petrol. Lead in paints has also been phased out and replaced by less harmful pigments. Most lead exposure now is likely to be from cheap imported toys and plastics or from plumbing in old houses where the tap-water is acid – a common problem in parts of Scotland. Lead is still used by some glass makers – be careful what you store in lead crystal decanters. Elsewhere, exposure to lead now is thought to be from historically contaminated land. This is most likely to affect you if you have an allotment on such a site. You can find out if there are problems by contacting your local environment agency and taking their advice on reducing your exposure.

The main source of cadmium is from smoking tobacco, and food and water from areas treated with sewage sludge and rock phosphate fertiliser used in intensive agriculture. Cadmium is also used as a bright orange pigment, including in some paints and expensive cooking pots, in nickel-cadmium (NiCad) batteries and in the electronics industries (especially for quantum computers). To avoid intake of cadmium, quit smoking, eat organic food and limit exposure to the other sources of the heavy metal; cook only in stainless steel or bamboo.

Some metals have been shown to have a beneficial effect on the brain. Lithium and rubidium, which are strongly alkaline metals, have been shown to increase levels of GABA and glutamic acid in the hypothalamus and amygdala, raising the possibility that mineral deficiencies might cause problems in some people.[41] Magnesium is also highly beneficial. There is more about this in Chapter 10, Food Factors 8 and 10.

Pesticides ('-cide' means 'killing')

Many pesticides are persistent organic pollutants and are increasingly implicated in neurological and mental illness. Strong links have been identified between pesticide use and Parkinson's, for example.[42]

The insecticides are of most concern. Many were developed at a time when it was thought that the nervous systems of insects and humans were different. It is now known that their nervous systems are closely similar: they even have identical DNA sequences.[43] Importantly, many insecticides can block receptors for GABA, the tranquillity neurotransmitter, with particular implications for anxiety disorders.

Organophosphate (OP) pesticides are of particular concern. They derive from the nerve gas that was developed by the Nazis during the Second World War and work by blocking the enzyme that normally breaks down the neurotransmitter acetylcholine after it has transmitted its 'move' message to muscles. As a result, nerves keep firing, leading in severe cases to over-stimulation, tremor and paralysis.

Until recently, organophosphates were used extensively in sheep dip to kill parasites such as those that cause sheep scab. Their use has been linked by some scientists and doctors to high suicide rates among hill farmers, although other factors such as social isolation may also have been important.[44] Organophosphates are also used as insecticides for the treatment of head lice in children and fleas in cats, dogs and other companion animals, and for infestations of insects in house plants and gardens.

Some of the effects of other groups of insecticides on the brain are summarised in the table below.

Sites of action on the nerve cells of some important insecticides

Substance	Effects
DDT Pyrethroids	Trains of false nerve impulses; tremors and other symptoms follow
Fipronil Lindane Cyclodienes	Inhibition of inhibitory signals with the potential for agitation and overactivity of some brain circuits
Nicotine Neonicotinoids Organophosphate insecticides Carbamates	Overstimulation, with tremor and paralysis

(modified from Stenersen)[45]

It can be seen that DDT and the synthetic pyrethroids can generate trains of false nerve impulses, causing tremors in serious cases. The organochlorine dieldrin, a persistent fat-soluble insecticide used in the past, is also known to affect neurotransmitter receptors in humans.

Unfortunately, patients are not normally tested for pesticides and other neurotoxic chemicals by their doctors or psychiatrists. Indeed, there is not even a standard protocol for testing them in the UK's National Health Service, so we have no idea what is the normal level of these substances in the body or what constitutes an abnormal level that could be a factor in the development of anxiety and depression. The Royal Commission on Environmental Pollution has recommended that a set of standard procedures for establishing people's levels of pesticides be developed and adopted, but this has yet to be implemented.[46] If you wish to find your own levels there are several laboratories that will perform such tests and tell you the likely implications (see Resources page 296). You can have your levels retested periodically to ensure the exposure reduction methods outlined below are working.

The best way of dealing with pesticides is to reduce exposure, so the body can start to eliminate them – and really detox!

A guide to detoxing

By following this list you can greatly reduce your exposure to potentially harmful chemicals.

- Buy as much organically produced food as possible. Eating organic can lower body burdens of pesticides in weeks. If you cannot afford to buy, try growing your own – even if this just means a few 'grow bags' on a balcony.

- Never buy chemicals that kill organisms in your home or garden. If some plant is going to die or have a few blotches on it, so be it. Once you stop poisoning things in your garden, nature will look after it for you – especially if you add lots of compost. Don't spray pesticides to treat house plants. If your pets have fleas, take them to the vet for an injection and then avoid their faeces. If your house has to be treated for an infestation, ensure that it is during warm weather so that you can ventilate it well afterwards. Use traditional methods of repelling insects, such as cedar wood or lavender to discourage moths. Love your spiders: they do an amazing job in reducing insect pests in the home and garden.

- Never buy cut flowers. Their perfect appearance reflects the fact that they have been doused in pesticides, destroying the ecosystems where they are produced and increasing pesticide levels when they are thrown away. Buy a pot plant or garden plant instead. Some hospitals now ban flowers because of the unnecessary work they create. A beautiful arrangement of organically produced fruit is much better for health and the environment.

- Unfortunately, many sports facilities such as golf courses or cricket pitches are kept looking perfect by the use of pesticides, and even a walk in countryside used for conventional arable agriculture or horticulture can expose us to pesticides. Try to avoid being there during or soon after spraying. If you live near to fields or amenities such as golf courses that are sprayed regularly, ask for prior notification of spraying and ensure that you keep doors and windows closed at such times.

- Keep your home well ventilated, especially if you have new carpets or curtains, or if you watch the television or work on a computer for any length of time. They are all likely to emit volatile chemical flame retardants. Also try to avoid breathing in fumes from paint, varnish or adhesives. Have lots of green house plants: they are good at removing toxic chemicals from the air in our homes.

- Try to avoid buying new cars. That new-car smell means you are breathing in a cocktail of volatile organic chemicals. Cars release yet more noxious chemicals as exhaust fumes, and the dust produced from tyres as they wear out contains some particularly nasty chemicals that end up as tiny particles that we can inhale. Walk or cycle whenever you can and use public transport instead of a car whenever possible.

- Fragrances, including sprays advertised for the lavatory or home or for the inside of cars, as well as those to be put on the skin, also contain man-made chemicals. All perfumes and fragrances are just chemical concoctions packaged and marketed to trick us into thinking that they somehow improve our image. Don't buy them! The clean smell of simple soap is much healthier and more attractive. Fresh lavender or other fresh flowers from your garden or a few pine leaves can smell wonderful.

- Try to use the simplest personal-care products such as natural crystal deodorants and baby shampoo. When you visit the hairdresser, try to avoid as many as possible of the chemical products on offer and never have your hair sprayed. Remember the old adage: if you wouldn't eat it don't put it on your skin or scalp! Use simple eco-friendly household cleaning products.

- Try to avoid using plastics. They can contain really damaging chemicals. Remember that the softer the plastic the more likely it is that toxic chemicals will leach out. Phthalates, which are used to soften plastics, can interfere with the neurotransmitter serotonin in the brain. Don't buy plastic toys for children, especially if they are likely to put them in their mouths. Use a metal pen or simple wooden pencil to write with. Have wooden or ceramic floors instead of plastic or man-made-fibre carpets.

- Use stainless steel, ceramics, heat-resistant glass and wooden spoons for cooking, and try to avoid using non-stick pans, microwave cookers or pressure cookers. Never dehydrate food between plastic sheets. Store food and drink in glass, earthenware or aluminium foil; this is much better than storing it in plastic.

- Finally, always wash your hands and rinse them thoroughly before eating.

Smoking

Tobacco smoke contains more than 200 toxic chemicals, including radioactive substances such as polonium-210, heavy metals such as cadmium, and hazardous organic chemicals such as the polycyclic aromatic hydrocarbons. If you are addicted to nicotine as a result of smoking and find it difficult to give up, you can reduce your risk by having nicotine patches or nicotine gum. It is the tar and smoke which cause health problems, not nicotine. If you do not smoke, try to avoid passive smoking, and if someone asks you if you mind if they smoke in your presence, just say 'Yes'.

Chapter Ten

The Ten Food Factors

THERE IS MOUNTING EVIDENCE that nutrition is vital to the brain and its proper functioning, and that the right kind of food can dramatically improve outcomes for people with mental illness.[1] The brain operates best when blood glucose is stable, which is best achieved by eating lots of complex carbohydrates and, in the long term, by consuming the types of fatty acids found in seafood. Research also confirms that eating breakfast is important to mental function in the morning. We give you ten easy-to-follow food factors to help you fight anxiety and depression.

A PROGRAMME, NOT A DIET

Lifestyle and health magazines and books are full of information about foods to fight depression, usually based on trying to boost serotonin levels. However, adding a few avocados or bananas to a diet full of saturated fat and chemical additives with too few nutrients is unlikely to help overcome depression or help with anxiety states. What is needed is a complete overhaul of eating habits to improve mental and physical well-being.

This might sound daunting, especially if you are feeling down, so here we give you ten simple food factors based on the latest scientific information, together with easy-to-follow tables to show you how to make the changes. Let us emphasise that this is a programme, not a diet. Diets, as many of us know from personal experience, don't work. They aren't much fun to follow and sooner or later we slide back to our old ways. Instead, our programme is flexible, allowing you to make sound choices.

Nutrition is especially important during pregnancy and breast-feeding to help prevent post-natal depression. It is particularly important to ensure an adequate intake of omega-3 fatty acids, vitamins and minerals (Food Factors 5 and 8).

Based on sound science

It is worrying that many of the books and articles on foods to fight depression are based on such poor science. For example, some people seem to think that patients with depressive illness who are often stressed and anxious need more noradrenaline. Indeed, noradrenaline has been referred to as 'the stress-busting chemical'.[2] In fact, it is often high levels of this neurotransmitter (relative to others, especially serotonin) that causes many of the distressing physical symptoms of depression, such as rapid heartbeat, panic attacks and insomnia. Indeed, beta blockers work by blocking the effects of noradrenaline on the heart.

In some diets we are advised to cut down on dairy (sometimes because of its links to heart disease, but with no information on what it does to the nervous system) but we may then be advised simply to change from hard cheese to hard sheep-milk cheese or from soft cheese to goat's cheese. Interestingly in our local supermarket one particular sheep-milk cheese highly recommended in one text is the most expensive cheese available: not much help to those off work as a result of ill health. Moreover, even after advising against dairy, books may include recipes full of dairy produce. The authors do not seem to know that all dairy products, especially hard cheese, have high levels of brain-damaging saturated fats which can make anxiety and depression worse.

We are often recommended to eat lots of oily fish as a good

source of essential omega-3 fatty acids needed for good brain function. This is bad advice because oily fish can contain high levels of pollutants that badly affect brain function. Hence the advice from the Food and Drug Administration in the USA and the Food Standards Agency in the UK is to limit fish to two portions a week of which only one should be oily fish (see page 199).[3] In fact, fish obtain their omega-3 fatty acids from the marine algae and plankton that they feed on and these can be bought in capsules, or you can obtain omega-3s from ultra-pure fish oils which have been processed to remove pollutants.

Changing diets, changing minds

As long ago as the 1970s, Professor Michael Crawford, a distinguished chemical nutritionist, warned that the explosion in the prevalence of heart disease that occurred throughout the West in the twentieth century would soon be followed by a similar increase in mental ill health.[4] At the time, there was great resistance to the idea that poor diets were contributing to the high rates of coronary heart disease, although now this seems almost a statement of the obvious and is accepted by even the most die-hard member of the medical establishment. A recent report entitled 'Changing diets, changing minds' states: 'We simply cannot wait another twenty years to reach the same position with food and mental health that it took to establish the link between poor diet and coronary disease.'[4] This report, which includes an excellent review of the state of our knowledge of dietary factors and their role in brain function, involved an impressive list of eminent scientists including nutritionists, behavioural scientists and psychiatrists. It follows an earlier survey on nutrition and health outcomes in the UK conducted by the leading British nutritionist Patrick Holford, and many other publications that had similar findings.[5] There is, in fact, an increasing consensus on what constitutes a healthy diet for the brain and mind. Interestingly, it is the same diet that helps to prevent and treat obesity, diabetes, heart disease and many types of cancer. *The Plant Programme*, which Jane wrote with Gill Tidey, is a cookbook which follows all the principles of such a healthy diet; it was designed particularly for cancer sufferers. *Eating for Better Health*, another book in the Plant Programme series, also contains many healthy, nutritious recipes ideal for people with anxiety and depression. The reason such knowledge about healthy diets never reaches most people is because of vested interests, including those of the food and pharmaceutical industries.[6]

But first let us look briefly at how this sorry picture of poor nutrition has come about in a society as rich and educated as ours. We are living longer, but this is often in a state of poor physical and mental health. It does not make sense that while most people are more prosperous than ever they are so poorly nourished that there is an explosion of physical and mental illnesses. Let us look in more detail at what has gone wrong with our food before considering what we can do about it.

Evolution and revolution

As we discussed in Chapter 3, the incredible flowering of the human brain occurred only about 200,000 years ago. In humans, the brain is the largest and hungriest organ in the body, consuming up to 70 per cent of all the calories we take in, about 20 to 30 per cent even when at rest. At the time the human brain evolved, our diet was very different to now. Indeed, many scientists think that many of our mental and physical health problems are caused by a diet that has changed beyond all recognition from the one eaten by early humans and the primates that preceded them.

As nature intended

For about 99 per cent of human and primate history, about 30 million years in all, our ancestors lived in small groups of hunter-gatherers, foraging for wild plants and animals. Their diet included edible roots, leaves, nuts, seeds, berries and other fruit, fish and shell fish, the meat of small animals, and occasionally meat from large mammals. Any animals killed were wild[7] and would themselves have had a diet mainly of fresh vegetables; all their organs would have been eaten, including the heart, liver and kidneys.[8] There were no dairy foods. A wide range of food was consumed[9] and it was eaten fresh. Overall calorie intake was low in relation to the energy expended in finding food.

Such a diet would have contained almost no saturated fats but lots of omega-3 and omega-6 essential fatty acids in the right proportions,[10] large quantities of carbohydrates, adequate protein and abundant vitamins and minerals.

Humans take control

Following the development of settled agriculture that began in the West about 10,000 years ago, the human diet became much more restricted. Cereals replaced fruit and vegetables as the main source of carbohydrates and there was a decrease in wild meat consumption.[11] About 8,000 years ago cows and other animals were domesticated and about 6,000 years ago milk began to be consumed in parts of southeast Europe and parts of Asia. The change to settled agriculture was accompanied by increased incidence of osteoporosis, dental caries and anaemia, and by reduced stature.[12]

Much later, and beginning in Britain in the seventeenth and eighteenth centuries, the agricultural and industrial revolutions led to further changes in our diet. The introduction of high-productivity agriculture, the mechanisation of food production and new preservation methods to feed the large number of workers in factories cheaply saw the beginnings of malnutrition unrelated to food shortages. White bread depleted in vitamins and minerals replaced wholemeal bread, and meat consumption increased dramatically. The malnutrition that resulted eventually led to the fortification of food with synthetic vitamins and minerals. Shipping produce around the world also meant that people began to eat old food preserved in alcohol, salt and sugar, often chemically denatured and altered.[13]

What we eat now

Data from the UK's national diet and nutrition survey shows that the UK diet is now dominated by cereals (predominantly refined wheat products) and meat and animal products, with much less fruit, vegetables and fish than during the Second World War.[14] Dairy is increasingly important in the Western diet, making up more than 40 per cent of the typical American diet. Alcohol consumption has increased dramatically, rising by about 20 per cent between 1990 and 2000, with many men and women now exceeding the recommended intake. Most dramatic of all has been the increase in fast and convenience foods. It has been estimated that the average person in the West eats over 4 kg of food additives every year. The amounts of additives in products are regulated based on advice from an expert committee of the Food and Agriculture Organisation and the World Heath Organisation (FAO/WHO), but serious concerns remain about their use.

Moreover, since the Second World War, we have used a huge range of chemical pesticides. Many have been banned when their damaging effects have been recognised, but about 350 are still used in conventional farming, and pesticides banned in the EU[15] such as DDT continue to be imported with imported food, flowers and other products.[16] The synthetic chemicals in pesticides and food additives are difficult, if not impossible, to test on animals for their mental-health effects.

As well as ingesting pesticides (many of which bioaccumulate up the food chain, becoming particularly concentrated in milk and meat fat) animals also ingest other harmful chemicals such as dioxins from industry and power generation and they are also treated with a wide range of veterinary products such as antibiotics and deworming agents and, in many countries, hormones. Increasingly, agriculture has been industrialised.

Why are we sick?

Clearly our diet is now dramatically different from that for which we and our brains have evolved. We now eat more food than our ancestors, but it is of a very limited range and it is lacking in nutrients. It contains too much saturated and trans fat, salt and refined white sugar and flour and too many synthetic chemicals from the agriculture and food-processing industries. Overall, our food is of poor quality, reflecting increasingly degraded soils, often treated with poisonous pesticides and other harmful substances, and it is rarely fresh having often been transported over great distances before it is eaten: typically it has travelled many 'food miles'.[17]

No wonder epidemiological research indicates that rates of depression rise as traditional diets are abandoned in favour of the Western diet.[18]

A revolution for our evolution

One of the reasons that the modern diet is associated with so many health problems is because human evolution is so slow compared to most other species on Earth. Just think about it! Bacteria live for only a few minutes – or hours at most – so that as individual bugs in a population are killed off by antibiotics, for example, those that are resistant survive to give us superbugs such as MRSA. In the 50 years since antibiotics were introduced, there will have been millions of generations of bugs but only about two generations of human beings. Clearly most of us will not have adapted to a diet that has changed as fast and as fundamentally as ours has, especially over the last 50 years. It follows that many of us are eating a diet that is totally unsuitable for human consumption. Interestingly, London Zoo used to have a notice asking people not to feed their food to animals because it would make them ill or kill them!

Let us now see what we can all do to improve our nutrition to help our mental health.

THE FOOD FACTORS

Our food factors are based on sound science. We know from our own experience and that of others that they can play an important role in improving both mental and physical well-being, and they can be used to develop a flexible healthy eating programme based on delicious meals – a regime that can be sustained. The ten food factors below, together with the ten lifestyle factors discussed in Chapter 9, comprise 'The Plant Programme for anxiety and depression', and some terrific recipes based on these principles are available in the cookbook *Eating for Better Health*. If you are using the Programme to prevent depression or prevent its return, we suggest that you incorporate the factors into your life at your own pace, proceeding from one to another when you feel ready. If you are suffering from mental illness now we suggest that you try to make the changes as quickly as possible. Before you begin, we think it is worth re-emphasising that just adding a few good foods to a diet that includes potentially harmful components will not help. For this reason, and as explained in Food Factor 2 below, we recommend that all the foodstuffs you consume should, as much as possible, be organically produced.

Let us now look at what dietary factors are needed to help the brain recover.

FOOD FACTOR 1: SOCIAL EATING

Boredom and loneliness frequently lead to depression, and anxiety can be much worse when there is nobody to share our worries with. Humans evolved as social animals, hunting, gathering, preparing and eating food in groups,[19] and countries where social eating is still important, such as those of southern Europe, have less depressive illness.

Preparing and eating food with others is a good way to start reconnecting with friends or family. So, depending on your circumstances, try to learn to make a few simple wholesome meals, ideally preparing them and eating with others. Cooking is a great way to increase your popularity and your social contacts. Simple vegetable soups, salads and baked potatoes are easy and provide good wholesome nutrition. So substitute them for sandwiches, burgers, pizzas and other processed food. If you are at present too ill or too low to make your own, buy them ready made from supermarkets or snack bars, making sure they don't contain any cheese, butter or margarine or spreads with trans fats or additives.

FOOD FACTOR 2: ORGANIC

Organic or biological agriculture is a system of food production that minimises the use of man-made chemicals. The emphasis is on the life cycle of the total environment, and organic food is generally fresh, live food.[20] Unfortunately most of our food is now produced by industrialised chemical agriculture with the liberal use of man-made fertilisers and pesticides. Farmed animals, including fish, are treated with a range of veterinary medicines such as antibiotics, deworming agents and, in many countries, hormones.[21] Individual cows now produce 39 pints of milk a day compared with 16 pints of milk a day in the 1970s.[22]

Chemical agriculture depletes soils of organic matter and of minerals such as calcium, copper, magnesium, iron, iodine, selenium and zinc, and the levels of these minerals are consequently low in the food produced from these soils.[23] At the same time, the use of chemical fertilisers such as superphosphates and nitrates increases the level of toxic substances such as cadmium and nitrates in the soil, and hence in our food and water. Pollution is increasing the levels of neurotoxic substances such as mercury and persistent organic pollutants, including pesticides, in soils and oceans globally.

There is increasing concern about the negative impact of pesticides on our emotional and mental well-being. The organic movement does use pesticides, but these tend to be natural substances whose anti-fungal or anti-insect properties are achieved by high concentrations. For example, high concentrations of copper sulphate may be used as a fungicide on crops, or high levels of salt may be used to kill sea lice on organically farmed fish. Copper sulphate and salt and the other pesticides used by the organic movement are all naturally occurring and are quite harmless when washed away and diluted. They are quite unlike the man-made molecules that make up artificial pesticides which do not exist in nature and can have unpredictable effects, sometimes at tiny concentrations.

Industrial chemical agriculture has made extensive use of synthetic pesticides since the Second World War, with successive families of chemicals being used and then phased out as the dangers to health were recognised. About 350 different pesticides are now used in conventional farming, with 31,000 tonnes sprayed annually in the UK alone.[24] Many pesticides that were formerly widely used, including some of the organochlorines such as DDT, aldrin and lindane, have now been banned in the EU and other Western countries, but they are still used in many tropical countries in which malaria is endemic and are contained in imported foods and other produce such as flowers.

Many insecticides are of particular concern because of their potential impact on the nervous system. As previously pointed out, at the time most pesticides were developed, it was assumed that the nervous system of insects was completely different to our own but we now know that the two systems are very similar, even down to their identical DNA sequences. The testing and regulation of pesticides is based on laboratory animals and cannot determine impacts on human mood and behaviour because of the difference between their brains and the human brain. Moreover, any cocktail effects of mixing different pesticides and other chemicals such as food additives are not identified.[25]

In 2002, almost 43 per cent of all vegetables and fruits tested in the UK contained pesticide residue, with some exceeding the approved limit.[26] Most of the produce, including 82 per cent of oranges tested by the Pesticides Residues Committee between 1998 and 2003, showed residues of multiple pesticides.[27]

Many pesticides that are now banned still persist in the environment, and they and other harmful chemicals from industry and power generation such as dioxins bioaccumulate or even bioconcentrate up the food chain, becoming particularly concentrated in animal fat, milk and fatty fish, especially farmed fish.[28] Much fish is contaminated with mercury, dioxins and PCBs, all of which can cause neurological and mental illness. Moreover in farmed fish the use of substances such as avermectin to control sea lice is of concern. Avermectins are fat-soluble, cross the blood–brain barrier and affect the activity of GABA, the tranquillity neurotransmitter, with the potential to worsen symptoms of anxiety. Avoid farmed oily fish and eat the fresh wild version instead. Otherwise, eat only white fish, ideally caught in areas that are relatively unpolluted such as Icelandic waters, and obtain your omega-3 essential fatty acids from purified cod liver oil. Mussels, including farmed mussels, from Scotland or Norway are ideal as sources of sea food and protein.

Food is frequently transported great distances before it is consumed and it may be up to four years old by the time it is eaten. This is of concern because the longer the time interval between harvesting and eating of food, the lower its nutrient content. This applies particularly to vitamins and natural enzymes which are easily lost through long storage and exposure of food to light, oxygen and heat. We try to avoid buying organic food flown in from other countries, because we cannot be sure it is truly organic, it is likely to be older than that from local farms, and flying such produce around the world makes pollution much worse. Moreover, such organic food may have been irradiated to increase its shelf life. Ideally buy locally grown organic food from farmers' markets.

A recent report by the National Consumer Council in the UK, entitled 'Greener?', shows that the best ratings for low pesticide residues and organic food in the UK were from Sainsbury's, Waitrose and Marks and Spencer.[29]

The good news is that changing to an organic diet significantly lowers the body burden of pesticides.[30]

FOOD FACTOR 3: ADDITIVES

There is a long history of using additives in the UK, developed from using salt, sugar, alcohol and vinegar to preserve food imported from the former colonies. Beginning in the industrial revolution, other chemicals began to be added to food in significant amounts and by the 1950s there was an explosion in the use of food additives, especially in the preparation of highly processed food and, more recently, convenience foods.

There has been a massive increase in the consumption of convenience foods, many of which are nutritionally poor compared to unprocessed wholefoods. They are typically high in empty calories, unhealthy saturated and trans fats, salt and refined carbohydrates and additives. There are approximately 320,000 different food and drink products on the market, with about 20,000 new ones introduced every year.[31] Moreover, the average person in the UK drank 186 litres of soft drinks in the year 2000 and now consumes nearly 44 kg of sugar a year.[32] In America, more than 20 billion tons of soft drinks are consumed every year.[33]

It has been estimated that at least 3,850 chemicals are now used as food additives in the manufacture of such convenience products, most of them chemically synthesised seasonings and flavourings.[34] Others are used to colour food to influence perceived flavour in anything from yoghurts to wine. Eric Schlosser, in his book *Fast Food Nation*, lists the more than 50 ingredients used to make the artificial strawberry flavour in a typical strawberry milk shake in the US. Other chemicals such as BHA, BHT and EDTA are commonly added to preserve foods and drinks. It has been suggested that BHT is toxic to the nervous system.

Some of the additives that are of particular concern for their potential effects on mental health are monosodium glutamate, aspartame[35] and tartrazine. Glutamate is manufactured in the body from protein, but we can take in excessively large amounts by consuming food that contains monosodium glutamate, usually known by its initials MSG.[35] Monosodium glutamate ('extra meaty flavour') is a major component of some soy sauces and many types of processed food.[35] It has been known to destroy nerve cells when fed to young animals, but some people maintain that it cannot cross the blood–brain barrier in human adults. The effectiveness of the blood–brain barrier relies on having the right kind of fat, and where the barrier is damaged or working imperfectly, MSG might increase agitation. MSG has been linked to dizziness, mood swings and depression.

The parts of the brain with NMDA receptors (see page 240) are particularly vulnerable to glutamate damage caused by excessive excitory activity, and it has been suggested that aspartate, aspartic acid, glutamate and glutamic acid, the 'acidic amino acids', which can be high in certain foods and drinks, are capable of destroying neurons when present in excessive amounts in the brain. Similarly, increased alertness or anxiety can be caused by the effect of caffeine in blocking receptors that normally inhibit glutamate release as well as its effects on GABA (the main inhibitory neurotransmitter) receptors.

There are currently 13 different types of man-made sugars, of which aspartame is the most widely used. Incredibly, artificial man-made sweeteners such as aspartame, made from wood alcohol, and saccharine made from petroleum, are classified as foods rather than flavourings. In 1985 Americans consumed 800 million pounds of aspartame, which is used in everything from diet drinks to yoghurts and chewing gum. Aspartame is currently being investigated because of suspicions about its links with brain tumours.[35] Other studies have linked it to headaches, depression, irritability, insomnia and effects on taste. It has also been linked to symptoms of anxiety, jitteriness and hyperactivity, so children with attention deficit hyperactivity disorder (ADHD) are recommended to avoid it.

Aspartame has three components: aspartic acid and phenylalanine, both of which can affect the balance of neurotransmitters in the brain, and methanol, which is an alcohol and a known neurotoxin and is generally coloured and flavoured to prevent it being consumed.

Tartrazine (E102, FD&C Yellow 5) is a synthetic yellow azo dye derived from coal tar and used as a food colouring. It can also be combined with E133 (brilliant blue) or E142 to produce various green shades (for tinned peas, for example). It is found in fruit squash and cordial, coloured soft drinks, instant puddings, cakes, custard, commercial soups and sauces, ice cream and lollies, sweets, chewing gum, jam and marmalade, mustard, yoghurt and many convenience foods. Amazingly, it is also found in some prescription drugs, including some antidepressants and over-the-counter medications, especially those containing glycerine, lemon and honey. And it is sometimes used to colour the capsules that pharmaceuticals such as antibiotics are contained in.

Tartrazine causes overactivity in children, especially where it is combined with benzoic acid (E210).[36] It also causes concentration and learning difficulties and depression, so we suggest that everyone with anxiety or depression should avoid this additive.

Although not normally an additive, caffeine in coffee or strong tea can lead to vitamin B deficiency, resulting in general anxiety.

Some processed food is labelled as organic, and if you are going to eat processed food this is probably the best, but ensure that it is frozen or packaged in a glass jar with a metal rather than a plastic lid and check the ingredients carefully for additives and ingredients such as refined sugar, salt and dairy before buying. Unfortunately the E number labelling system used in the EU does not allow any distinction to be made between harmful chemicals and those that are relatively benign.

FOOD FACTOR 4: BALANCING THE DIET TO IMPROVE MOOD

A person's food intake affects brain function and hence mood and behaviour. Just think how irritable and restless or apathetic and moody you can become when you are hungry. Surges in blood sugar that are followed by lows, can cause stress hormones such as cortisol to rise and cause massive mood swings. Simply changing your diet to prevent this happening can greatly reduce your stress levels. Often it is the complex interaction of nutrients rather than a single nutrient that is needed to improve brain function, and the balance of protein, carbohydrates and fats in the diet, as well as the intake of vitamins and minerals, is particularly important.

In the UK and the US and many other developed countries, alcoholism, drug taking and fad diets are responsible for the bulk of nutritional deficiencies that can affect mental functioning.[37] In the case of fad diets, high-protein diets such as Dr Atkins' 'New Diet Revolution' and 'Protein Power' are of particular concern. The recent craze for 'low-carb' diets such as the Atkins' Diet may have been beneficial to the financial interests of the meat and dairy industries, but it has been very damaging for health. The basis of low-carb diets is that if carbohydrate intake is low the body will be forced to burn fat and protein as fuels. As some nutritionists have pointed out, this is like burning the fabric of your house or your antique furniture instead of firewood to provide heat or energy. If this goes on for any length of time the fabric of the house will become seriously weakened. In the same way the use of low-carb diets mean that the muscles in our bodies will break down and our bones will also be weakened, giving rise to osteoporosis and other bone diseases. T. Colin Campbell, perhaps the world's greatest nutritional scientist, has discussed the many health problems of such diets. He concludes with reference to the Atkins' Diet that 'it is a testament to the power of modern marketing savvy that an obese man with heart disease and high blood pressure (Dr Atkins) became one of the richest snake oil salesmen ever to live.'[38]

Let us remind ourselves that we evolved as a species eating masses of unrefined carbohydrates for energy, a little fat as an energy store and for warmth, and protein mainly from plant sources for the growth and repair of our bodies. The diet traditionally eaten by rural Chinese people follows the same principles and provides a good basis for a healthy balanced diet. A team of international scientists from Cornell University in the US, Oxford University in the UK and Beijing University in China reported in the 1980s on the enormous health benefits of this diet.[38]

Experimental studies clearly show the negative impacts of low-carbohydrate diets on mood.[38] Animal experiments all show that animals fed high-carbohydrate diets are healthier in every way. They live longer, are more physically active and are slimmer. Animals kept on low-carbohydrate high-protein diets, especially those high in dairy protein, are sluggish and quickly show signs of fatigue.[38] Human studies give similar results. One experiment on trained female cyclists, for example, showed significantly greater tension, depression, anger and a lower total mood score in those on a low-carbohydrate diet than those on a high-carbohydrate diet.[39]

The correct balance of foods in our diet also influences how acid or alkaline our blood can become, which can in turn affect how our bodies and our minds behave.[40] If we eat too much protein, especially animal protein, the blood becomes too acid and we become lethargic and depressed. Interestingly, hard cheese is the most acid-generating food in the Western diet,[41] about three times as acid-generating, weight for weight, as roast beef.[42] We know of several people who were profoundly depressed and who were surviving on cheese in various forms, often cheese sandwiches. Once cheese was banished and their diet rebalanced, they recovered fully.

If you are well, you should aim for a diet that is 60 per cent alkaline-generating foods and 40 per cent acid-generating foods. If you are ill, you should try to increase your alkaline-generating food to about 80 per cent of your diet – but beware! There is a lot of misleading information about which foods generate acidity and alkalinity in the body. For reliable information based on sound scientific research, go to www.janeplant.com or the charts in Jane's book *Eating for Better Health*.

FOOD FACTOR 5: FATS

In Chapter 2 we discussed how the brain comprises 60 per cent fat, which is essential for its structure and function. The importance of fat in the brain is strongly made by Hibbeln, a psychiatrist from the National Institutes of Health in the US who is quoted as saying 'One day I was standing in my lab, holding a human brain in my hand, and it suddenly hit me, the brain is all fat. There is no difference between your brain and a stick of butter.'[43]

Saturated fats

This is a very important observation – although likening the brain to a stick of butter is unfortunate because butter is almost entirely saturated fat which is bad for brain function; it just clogs it up and stops it working. As we shall discover, the brain needs only the right kind of fats, but the Western diet contains far too much bad saturated fat, mainly from meat and dairy products.[44] In the UK many dairy products, including cheese, butter and full-fat yoghurts (now often called probiotics), are now classed as junk food by the Food Standards Agency because of the amount of unhealthy saturated fats they contain.

The problem has become much worse because animals are kept in industrial battery pens and prevented from exercising, and they are fed cereals or soya rather than grass or fresh vegetables.[45] Intensively reared animals now have significantly higher ratios of saturated fat to quality protein than wild species. The amount of saturated fat in chickens has increased from 2 per cent in wild birds to 22 per cent in battery chickens.[46] The amount of saturated fat in intensively reared cattle is 30 per cent, compared with 5 per cent in the wild species.[47] Farmed fish have much higher levels of fat than the same species in the wild,[48] with higher levels of omega-6 essential fatty acids (EFAs) relative to omega-3 EFAs.

Trans fats

The manufacture of processed foods – including cakes, pastries, biscuits and products from fast food outlets – introduced hydrogenated fats, known as 'trans' fats, into our diet. These are manufactured using industrial processes that make vegetable oils solid at room temperature and were introduced to give products a long shelf life. The 'trans' refers to a special type of chemical bond in the molecules called 'trans bonds'. They are bad fats because when we eat them the body treats them as just fats, but they inhibit the enzymes that convert simple omega-3 and omega-6 oils into the long-chained versions needed for brain structure and function.[49] They have no nutritional value and many food agencies are now warning of their potential harmful effects. Many margarines and spreads now state how much trans fat they contain and it is possible to choose ones that have very low levels.

Essential fats

The two types of fats essential for brain function are the omega-6 and omega-3 essential fatty acids (EFAs).[49] Linoleic acid (LA) is the simplest

Dietary Sources of Fats

Saturated fats: eliminate** or reduce*	Trans-fatty acids (TFAs): eliminate	Monounsaturated fats: 'Good fats'	Polyunsaturated fats: 'Good fats'
Butter**	Margarine	Olives and olive oil	Vegetable oils
Cheese**	Cooking fats	Almonds	Sesame seeds and oil
Milk**	Cakes	Pecan nuts	Safflower seeds and oil
Red meats*	Highly processed foods, such as some commercial mayonnaise, dressings and creams	Peanuts	Sunflower seeds and oil
Fatty poultry such as duck*		Cashew nuts	Corn oil
Coconut oil*		Walnuts	Wheat-germ oil
Margarine**		Fish	Flax oil
Palm oil*			Pecan nuts
			Pine nuts
			Evening primrose oil
			Soya oil and beans
			Cold-water fish and fish-liver oils

omega-6 EFA, from which other more complex long-chained polyunsaturated fatty acids (LC-PUFA) such as gamma-linoleic acid and arachidonic acid can be synthesised. LA is termed essential because the body cannot make it so it must be obtained from the diet. Vegetable oils such as sunflower and soya oils are particularly rich sources.

Similarly, the simplest omega-3 EFA, alpha-linoleic acid (ALA), must be consumed as part of the diet – from nuts and seafood, for example. It has been suggested that the human brain could not have evolved without access to large omega-3 resources from shellfish and other seafoods.

ALA can be converted into other LC-PUFAs including eicosapentaenoic acid (EPA) and docosahexaenoic acid (DHA) in the body, but this process can be ineffective in some people. The LC-PUFAs such as DHA are especially important for the brain. Without them, cell membranes, instead of being fluid, become rigid and less flexible, with abnormal functioning of receptors so that communication between neurons is impaired. There are genetic differences between individuals in their ability to convert simple omega-3s and omega-6s into the vital LC-PUFAs. The synthesis of LC-PUFAs in the body is also badly affected and even prevented by the presence of saturated fats and trans fats, stress hormones (see further under Lifestyle Factor 1, page 176) and alcohol. Mineral and vitamin deficiencies, as well as many types of viral infections, can also prevent the synthesis of LC-PUFAs.[49]

Another problem that stems from our poor diet is that the proportion of omega-6 to omega-3 EFAs has changed dramatically. Most of us eat too little of the omega-3 EFAs.[50] It has been estimated that our diet now contains 16 times as much omega-6 as omega-3 EFAs, whereas a century ago the amounts would have been about equal. Hibbeln has reported that levels of serotonin, the feel-good neurotransmitter in the brain, increase as omega-3 EFAs increase in the diet, while overall blood flow in the brain and the growth of brain cells, axons and dendrites improves with increasing DHA intake.[50] It may also protect brain cells from damage or dying, which can happen in conditions of chronic stress. There is also mounting epidemiological and clinical evidence, including evidence from brain imaging, that increasing omega-3 EFAs in the diet can help prevent and treat depression, even in cases where drugs such as Prozac have proved ineffective.[50]

The suggestion of a link between the type of fat in the diet and depression has been confirmed by several studies. Professor Basant Puri, of the Imaging Sciences Department, Hammersmith Hospital, part of Imperial College, London, has produced compelling evidence that the fat profile of the diet is crucial for mental health, including that of children.[51] Studies in Israel showed improvements in patients with depression within two weeks of taking fish oil high in EPAs.[52] After four weeks, 60 per cent of those taking the fish oil had a 50 per cent decrease in symptoms such as insomnia or feelings of worthlessness. Only one in ten patients in the placebo group reported similar improvements. In another study at Sheffield University, large doses of omega-3 EFAs were given to 70 depressed patients who had failed to respond to Prozac treatment. At 12 weeks, 60 per cent of the patients showed marked improvement, compared with 25 per cent of the control group given placebos.[52] The good thing about taking extra omega-3 EFAs is that, unlike antidepressants, they have no side effects.

As a result of these findings, many authors writing popular books and articles are busy telling us to eat loads of oily fish, but there are several reasons why this is bad advice.

- In order to obtain adequate levels of EPA, a very large amount of fish would have to be consumed. About 400 g of fresh tuna each day, for example.[53]

- Fish is now heavily contaminated with neurotoxic metals, especially mercury, lead and cadmium, as well as dioxins and PCBs, which are linked to cancer. Hence the American FDA and the UK FSA have issued a warning to pregnant mothers not to consume more than the equivalent of about half a can of tuna a week, which is about 300 g.

- Ultra-purified fish oils are readily available.

- Fish obtain their good omega-3 fatty acids from the marine algae they eat, and these can be bought in capsules (which are also suitable for vegans).[54]

Ten ways to improve your brain fats

If you used to do this...	Now do this!
Eat butter or spreads full of trans fats on bread, toast and sandwiches	Drizzle a little organic extra virgin olive oil on your savoury sandwiches instead, or spread them with humus
Cook with unspecified vegetable oil or, worse still, lard, butter or margarine	Grill or steam whenever possible. Cold-pressed extra virgin olive oil is the most stable oil when heated, so use it for everything from stir-fries to fried potatoes
Snack on cakes, biscuits, chocolates	Read all labels and avoid foods high in saturated and trans fats. Substitute with mezzos dipped into humus or taramasalata. Keep little packets of nuts and dried fruit to snack on
Eat cheese-laden pizza from your take-away	Ask for a marguerite with no mozzarella and have extra olives, capers, mushrooms, peppers, artichokes and aubergines instead
Eat lots of factory-farmed chicken, pork, bacon or beef or, worse still, sausages laden with saturated fat from animals prevented from exercising	Eat organic free-range meat or wild game and only in moderation. Wild venison and wild rabbit are particularly good
Treat yourself to cheesy hamburgers in white-bread buns	Instead buy some delicious fish or vegetable sushi or a lunch box from a supermarket, or, better still, a Japanese, Korean or Chinese shop
Eat loads of saturated-fat-packed ice cream, cheese, butter, milk and yoghurt	Dump the dairy completely and use soya, rice, oat or other vegetable substitutes for milks, creams, yoghurt and ice cream. Buy delicious pre-marinated or smoked tofu to substitute for cheese

If you used to do this…	Now do this!
Pile bought mayonnaise, salad cream or other glop on your salads	Learn to make a few delicious salad dressings. Just add one part wine vinegar to two parts olive or sunflower oil with a squeeze of fresh lemon as your base. Add black pepper, garlic and fresh herbs to taste
Eat bought breakfast cereals with lashings of milk and white sugar	Make some organic porridge; add some stewed fruit and a dash of soya or rice milk for a delicious brain-healthy start to the day
Think a good breakfast means fried eggs, bacon, sausages and black pudding	Eat a grilled kipper or a small piece of haddock poached in soya milk and water. Add a slice of lemon and a poached egg if you wish

FOOD FACTOR 6: FUELLING UP ON CARBOHYDRATES

Carbohydrates and energy supply

As we learned in Food Factor 4, we need large amounts of carbohydrates (starches and sugars) in our diet because these, not protein or fat, are the ideal foods for energy supply including for the brain. Complex carbohydrates such as wholemeal bread or pasta are particularly helpful in maintaining a steady supply of glucose to the brain. Carbohydrates also significantly affect mood and behaviour because eating a meal high in carbohydrates triggers the release of insulin in the body. Insulin helps blood sugar to enter cells where it can be used for energy. Also, as insulin levels rise, more tryptophan, the precursor of serotonin, enters the brain. The higher serotonin levels in the brain enhance mood and have a sedating effect, so people often feel pleasantly calm and drowsy after a meal high in carbohydrates. Tryptophan deficiency is known to aggravate premenstrual tension.[55]

On the other hand, when blood sugar falls because we are hungry or because we have hypoglycaemia from eating a bad diet with too many refined carbohydrates (see below), not only do levels of feel-good chemicals fall but the stress hormones adrenaline and cortisol are released.

Bad carbohydrates

Unfortunately, many people crave bad carbohydrates. Eating these can cause rapid swings in blood sugar (and hence in mood) and they are generally considered bad for both mental and physical health.[56] Indeed, it has been suggested that some cases of depression are related entirely to problems caused by eating such foods.

It is always worth remembering that as long ago as 1972 white sugar was described as 'pure, white and deadly' by Professor Yudkin, the famous Cambridge biochemist.[57] Thirty-five or more years later it is still added to many convenience foods and snacks. Bad carbohydrates include any foods containing refined white starch, refined white sugar, polished white rice or other refined white cereals – including that extracted from potatoes and turned into junk food snacks known in the trade as 'extruded starch food products'. Refined carbohydrates are just empty calories, depleted of vital vitamins, minerals and enzymes, since these are removed in processing – for example in the extraction of white sugar (sucrose) from sugar cane or sugar beet.

For the body to digest and use such foods, the missing minerals, vitamins and enzymes must be found from somewhere else in the body, leading to depletion in vital nutrients and often making us feel even hungrier as our body signals to us to replace the missing nutrients.[58]

Good carbohydrates

There are many good carbohydrate foods, especially fruit and vegetables, the energy foods we evolved to eat.[59] As well as some calories, these foods are packed with healthy antioxidants, vitamins and minerals, fibre, live enzymes and other good-for-health phytochemicals – so eat as many as you can, as raw and fresh as possible.[60] Drink fresh juices and have loads of salads, vegetable soups and lightly steamed or stir-fried vegetables.

Other good starches include wholegrain cereals, bread and pasta, and brown rice. Root vegetables, such as potatoes (particularly with their jackets on), are especially good.

We evolved with a liking for sweet foods, and fruit is especially good for those with a sweet tooth. Other good sources of sugar include molasses, raw unrefined sugar (not white sugar that has been dyed brown) and raw unpasteurised honey and maple syrup.

Ten ways of fuelling up on good carbohydrates

If you used to do this...	Now do this!
Wake up with coffee or tea with milk and white sugar	Substitute green tea with freshly squeezed lemon, lime or orange and a dash of honey to taste, and repeat this throughout the day
Breakfast on packet cereals fortified with added vitamins, fibre and minerals, with lashings of white sugar and dairy milk	Make some porridge with raw organic oats and add some fruit stewed in a little orange juice and raw brown sugar for a delicious healthy start to the day
Eat loads of biscuits with sugary coffee at elevenses	Have herbal or green tea and munch on a wholegrain cereal or sesame bar
Snack on sweets, candies and cakes all day, especially when you are bored	Try freshly shelled nuts or dried fruit instead, or eat apples, bananas or pears
Grab a white-bread sandwich or baguette for lunch	Eat a baked potato filled with humus or baked beans instead (but try to avoid those that contain hidden sugar). Accompany with a freshly made salad with a tasty vinaigrette dressing
Munch on potato crisps or other starchy potato snacks made with reconstituted starch, or a sesame bar flavoured with chemical additives	Eat the odd bag of organic lightly salted real crisps or, better still, unsalted nuts

If you used to do this...	Now do this!
Drink loads of fizzy, sugary colas, squashes and fruit drinks	Substitute fresh veggie juices, fruit juices and smoothies. There are some delicious recipes for juices and smoothies in *Eating for Better Health*
Eat lots of white pasta or pizza	Buy the wholegrain version and eat with home-made tomato sauces and loads of freshly steamed or lightly stir-fried vegetables
Buy loads of white rice to eat with your take-away	Have fried brown rice instead, and, better still, make your own sauce
End your meals with sugary starchy puddings and ice cream	Base your puds on fruit. Eat lots of fruit salads and baked or stewed fruit with soya ice cream or home-made lemon or orange sorbet

FOOD FACTOR 7: PROTEINS, THE GOOD, THE BAD AND THE DANGEROUS

The first thing to say about protein is that in the West we generally eat far too much of it. An adequate supply of protein in the diet is important for maintaining and repairing the structure of cells, especially if they are being damaged by, for example, overdosing on alcohol or drugs, but it is quite unsuitable for energy generation. It is estimated that only 5 to 6 per cent of our daily calorie intake should be protein to replace that excreted by our bodies, with a maximum intake of only about 10 to 11 per cent.[61] Many in the West consume much higher levels – up to 15 to 16 per cent – and some people eat an unhealthy 20 per cent or more. Certainly this is true of some fad diets such as the low-carbohydrate diets promoted by Dr Atkins.[61] In contrast, the traditional Chinese diet typically contains less than 11 per cent protein of which only about 1 per cent is animal protein.

There are eight essential amino acids that the body cannot synthesise itself and must be supplied by the diet. Meat, fish, eggs and soya contain the complete range, but you can also get the complete range by combining different plant proteins such as cereals and pulses. The traditional Jamaican dish of rice and peas provides a complete range of protein, for example, and so does the traditional Mexican dish of beans wrapped in a tortilla.

Protein intake can affect brain functioning and mental health. Some of the brain's important neurotransmitters are made from amino acids. For example, the neurotransmitter dopamine is made from the amino acid tyrosine, and serotonin is synthesised from tryptophan. If there is too little of the precursor amino acid in the body there will be too little of the neurotransmitter in the brain, resulting in low mood and depression. However, too much protein competes with the transport of the amino acid precursors, especially tryptophan, to the brain. As usual, then, the guiding principle here is one of balance between insufficient intake of vital amino acids and overdosing on too much protein. It is always a good idea to minimise the amount of high-protein foods, especially animal foods, we eat before trying to sleep.

Ideally for health, most of the protein in our diet should be from plant, not animal, sources.[62] There is no doubt that hypertension (high blood pressure) and high blood cholesterol are bad for the brain. These conditions reflect diets too high in animal products, usually eaten as a source of protein. The main culprits are meat and dairy, especially products from industrialised farms and eggs from battery chickens. High intakes of animal protein in the absence of adequate vegetables and fruit in the diet can lead to the formation of damaging oxidising chemicals such as homocysteine in the body. This is now being linked to brain damage leading to dementia. Most meat and cheese, in addition to any protein they contain, are full of saturated fat from animals fed grain-rich diets on factory farms. Animal-based foods not only activate free-radical production that causes cell damage in the brain and elsewhere, but they also lack antioxidants.[63] On the other hand, plant-based protein from nuts, seeds, grains and pulses are full of brain-healthy antioxidants, vitamins and minerals and they contain no cholesterol.

Ten ways of having healthy proteins

If you used to do this...	Now do this!
Think cooked breakfast means bacon, eggs, sausages and black pudding	Try 'bubble and squeak' – potato and cabbage or other previously cooked veg, fried in olive oil with lots of black pepper
Always have at least two hard-boiled eggs a day	Have one a day max, and lightly poach it instead. Substitute a grilled tomato for the second egg
Think steak (cow) pie and chips is a good pub lunch	Order fish and chips instead, or a baked potato with salad
Always lunch on a cheese-and-pickle sandwich	Try humus and roast or grated veg instead, with a delicious dressing
Have lots of chicken or meaty soups	Make delicious vegetable or miso soups. Add split peas or lentils for protein and eat with cubes of toasted wholemeal bread
Think supper means chicken or a pork chop	Have an omelette packed with vegetables (but not if you have a daily breakfast egg) or a dish with brown rice and beans
Eat lots of take-away meaty curries	Learn to make simple curries yourself and then add chunky vegetables such as cauliflower, broccoli or tofu
End every dinner party with cheese	Keep to four courses and add a couple of delicious salads or salsas between the soup and the main dish
Think Sunday lunch means a large roast with two veg	Cook a much smaller roast and increase the veg. Add caramelised onions in red wine, carrots with garlic and white wine, at least two types of green veg, steamed minted potatoes, and potatoes roasted in olive oil

If you used to do this...	Now do this!
Eat animal protein at every meal	Eat just one small portion of animal protein a day. Choose from grilled fish, lightly cooked egg dishes or wild or free-range meat

FOOD FACTOR 8: VITAMINS, MINERALS AND SUPPLEMENTS

Vitamins

Many vitamins and minerals are essential co-factors in making the chemicals needed for optimum brain function. They are involved in the synthesis of neurotransmitters from precursor chemicals, for example. Many conditions caused by vitamin and mineral deficiencies (including scurvy caused by vitamin C deficiency, or anaemia caused by iron deficiency) are associated with depressed mood; indeed, psychological change is frequently the first symptom of such conditions. Here are some notes about the most important vitamins and minerals for mental health.

Vitamin A

Deficiency or excess of vitamin A can cause headaches and feelings of increased pressure in the head. Excess can also cause fatigue, irritability and loss of appetite. Good sources of vitamin A include meat, fish, eggs, orange vegetables and green, leafy vegetables.

The B vitamins

These are water-soluble and any excess is generally excreted safely from the body. But they can leach from food during cooking.

Folic acid (folate), unlike the other B vitamins, is readily stored in the liver. Good dietary sources include leafy green vegetables, pulses (peas, beans and lentils), yeast, mushrooms, nuts and whole grains. It helps prevent the formation of homocysteine during the metabolism of methionine.

Vitamin B1 (thiamine) is essential for the metabolism of glucose, the brain's main food. Sources include tuna and lentils. It can become deficient in people who habitually drink strong coffee or tea, resulting in symptoms of fatigue, general anxiety and even agoraphobia. Alcohol also causes deficiency of this vitamin with serious consequences in cases of abuse. Alcoholics show a lower mean serum concentration of vitamin B1, with or without a decrease of folate or vitamin B12. Vitamin B1 deficiencies, which often occur in alcoholics, can cause severe neurological problems such as impaired movement and memory loss. The neurological damage is called Wernicke's encephalopathy,[64] while the resulting memory damage (which leads the sufferer to tell often inextricable lies in response to questions, a condition known as confabulation) is Korsakoff's syndrome.[65] Causes of thiamine deficiency in alcoholics are insufficient dietary intake, inhibition of intestinal absorption and reduced storage in the liver due to disease.

Vitamin B3 (niacin or nicotinic acid) can be made in the liver from the amino acid tryptophan. Good dietary sources include pulses, wholegrain cereals, nuts, meat and fish. Deficiencies are associated with predominantly corn or maize diet, alcoholism or drug abuse associated with malnutrition and some pharmaceutical treatments. Severe deficiency causes pellagra which is associated with serious neurological symptoms such as seizures, fits and psychosis. It is important to realise that deficiency in just this one B vitamin can lead to psychosis.

Vitamin B6 (pyridoxine) is another important vitamin for the brain and nervous system.[66] The food additive tartrazine can lead to a deficiency of vitamin B6, as can some antidepressants. Vitamin B6 deficiency is characterised by mental changes such as fatigue, nervousness, irritability, depression and insomnia, related to the body's inability to manufacture some neurotransmitters as a result of this deficiency. Unfortunately, excess vitamin B6 (more than 500 mg per day) can cause nerve damage. Good dietary sources include wholegrain cereals, leafy green vegetables, pulses, fruit, eggs, meat and fish.

Vitamin B12 contains the trace element cobalt. Ruminant herbivorous animals such as cows and sheep obtain theirs by ingesting soil which contains microbes which make vitamin B12. In the past, people probably had a similar supply,[67] but the use of pesticides (which means that food must be thoroughly cleaned) and the general obsession with hygiene means that micro-organisms may no longer be an adequate source for humans. We suggest you buy organically produced vegetables (not imported organic food, which may have been irradiated to kill off any microbes), wash them only in cold water and eat some raw. The microbes will increase in your gastro-intestinal tract and keep you supplied with B12, but beware of killing them off with antibacterial products, drugs, alcohol or medicine (especially antibiotics). Other good dietary sources include meat and brewer's yeast.

'Vitamin' B8 Inisotol may be classified as a member of the vitamin B complex, although it is not strictly a vitamin itself. Supplementation has been found to be helpful in bulimia, panic attacks and bipolar disorder. It is especially high in unrefined cereals, nuts, beans and fruit, especially cantaloupe melons, bananas and oranges, as well as unrefined molasses and brewer's yeast. Coffee destroys this nutrient.

Vitamin C

Vitamin C is essential. One of its roles is as an antioxidant – important for the whole nervous system. The famous scientist Linus Pauling (winner of two Nobel prizes) recommended that we take at least a gram a day of vitamin C, whereas most government-recommended doses are less than a tenth of that. Pauling's recommendation was based on his calculation of the amount of vitamin C consumed by gorillas in the wild eating an essentially vegan diet. Unfortunately, this has led to many people taking a gram of *synthetic* vitamin C a day. The real message is to eat masses of fresh raw fruit and vegetables. Citrus fruits, all berries, green apples, melons, pineapples and kiwi fruit are good sources, as well as green vegetables, tomatoes, peppers and root vegetables such as potatoes and turnips. Vitamin C levels in produce fall during storage and can be lost as a result of cooking in water, especially if sodium bicarbonate is used or if you cook in copper pans.

Vitamin D

Vitamin D deficiency has been linked to depression and it has been suggested that it is a factor in seasonal affective disorder (SAD) because it is normally made in the skin by the action of sunlight. Good dietary sources include fish and fish oils, but beware because excessively high levels also cause depression.

Vitamin E

This is the major fat-soluble antioxidant in the body, and depression has been shown to be accompanied by low levels in the blood. It is particularly important in relation to maintaining the brain's fats in a healthy state. Vitamin E deficiency causes nerve tissues to degenerate, with symptoms of dizziness, visual and other sensory changes which, if untreated, can become irreversible. Good sources of vitamin E include nuts, seeds, wholegrain unrefined cereals, plant oils and green, leafy vegetables.

Vitamin H (biotin, coenzyme R)

Vitamin H deficiency is linked to depression. Good dietary sources include wholegrain cereals (especially brown rice), nuts, fruit, yeast and cooked eggs. Deficiencies are associated with eating raw eggs, which contain a protein that prevents biotin absorption.

Minerals

Mineral deficiencies can cause a variety of medical conditions, from night blindness to skin lesions, and in some cases they can inhibit the synthesis and function of neurotransmitters in the brain. We first consider lithium because of its known use in treating bipolar disorder and the latest evidence that modern diets may be deficient in this element. It also exemplifies many of the problems in ensuring we have the correct balance of minerals in our diet.

Lithium

Like many other trace elements that are considered essential for man and animals, lithium can be so deficient in our diet that biological function is impaired, or so high that toxicity occurs and damage is caused (for this reason blood levels are carefully monitored when it is used clinically to treat bipolar disorder). There is a range of concentrations between these extremes in which function is optimal.[68] The reason such high doses of lithium are needed to treat bipolar disorder should be questioned. As discussed on page 176, this is likely to reflect difficulties in sodium ions crossing cell membranes. This problem is now considered by many distinguished biochemists, doctors and neuroscientists to reflect rigidity of cell walls, because we have too little of the essential fatty acids in our diet (see page 222 above).[69]

Apart from people with bipolar disorder on medication, there is little likelihood of lithium toxicity but there is much evidence that our intakes may be too low as a result of using reprocessed water, growing crops using intensive agriculture and a decline in the consumption of seafood. Lithium deficiency in experimental animals has been shown to increase levels of stress hormones (as well as leading to the development of ovarian cysts and mammary gland problems). The behaviour of lithium-deficient rats is characterised by lower physical activity, decreased pleasure in being handled and lower assertiveness in interactions with rats on lithium-adequate diets. Evidence published in 1991 links low lithium intakes with altered behaviour and aggressiveness in humans and shows that low lithium levels are associated with increased numbers of mental hospital admissions. Statistically significant associations between low lithium levels and suicide, murder, rape and possession of drugs have also been reported. Lithium supplementation studies have shown that the element improves mood scores. A provisional RDA (recommended daily allowance) of 1 mg a day is recommended for adults, and this can normally be provided by diet, though people on dialysis and with certain diseases may still be deficient. Growing children, adolescents and mothers who are breast feeding may need more than the RDA.

Lithium can be obtained from natural spring or stream water in some areas, but its levels in crops reflects the lithium content of the underlying soils and rocks. New geochemical maps of Europe show that lithium levels in water vary by a factor of 3,600 times, (from 0.1 µg l^{-1} in northern Europe over Norway, Sweden and Finland up to 360 µg l^{-1} around the Mediterranean in Spain and Italy). In the UK, levels are highest over England and lower over Scotland, Wales and Northern Ireland. A more rigorous analysis is needed, but it is interesting that lithium levels are lowest in countries with the highest rates of suicide, according to the World Health Organisation.[70]

Seafood is the most reliable source, and we particularly recommend sea vegetables as a source; see Food Factor 4 above.

Zinc

Zinc is important for mental alertness, taste and smell. Zinc deficiency can cause depression, loss of appetite, poor wound healing, hair loss and impaired taste and smell. Deficiency is often associated with white spots on the fingernails. The food additive tartrazine can lead to a deficiency of zinc. Good dietary sources include red meat, liver, eggs, some seafoods (especially oysters), wholegrain cereals, pulses, seeds (especially pumpkin seeds) and yeast.

Selenium

Selenium is an essential antioxidant and it also plays a vital role in maintaining good thyroid function. Selenium toxicity causes changes in the nervous system associated with fatigue and irritability. Good dietary sources include seafood, liver and eggs; also grain and seeds, but this depends on the selenium state of the soil.

Copper

Copper is involved in iron metabolism in the body and in brain function. Deficiency causes anaemia, with inadequate oxygen supply to the brain, decreased levels of neurotransmitters and changes in their receptors. The best dietary sources include organ meats, seafood, nuts, seeds, wholegrain bread and cereals, and chocolate.

Magnesium

Magnesium is involved in the transmission of nerve impulses. Deficiency can cause agitation and nervousness, twitching and unsteadiness. Serious deficiency can cause delirium and convulsions. Good sources include green leafy vegetables, wholegrain cereals, nuts, seeds and bananas.

Other important minerals for the brain and nervous system include iodine (from seafood), chromium (from brewer's yeast and black pepper), iron (from meat, green leafy vegetables, and dried beans, peas and fruit), calcium (from salmon, sardines and dark green leafy vegetables) and manganese (wholegrain cereals and nuts).

Supplements

Nutritional supplements should be used with great care because some, like vitamin A, can result in an overdose, especially where there is liver damage, and excess vitamin D can actually cause depression. Supplementation over a period of time can also cause other health problems such as increased blood pressure.

The best way to treat dietary deficiencies is to eat an adequate diet and generally we advise against man-made vitamin and mineral pills. All good recent nutritional research indicates that for our bodies to be able to use vitamins and minerals effectively they need to be in a food our body can recognise, not in a pill containing more man-made chemicals.[71] However, the following supplements are very helpful for preventing and treating depression.

Ultra-pure fish oils

These contain vitamins A and D and LC-PUFAs. Vegans can take capsules of marine algae such as those called 'eau plus', marketed by a Swiss company, which contain the vital LC-PUFAs. Dark-green leafy vegetables are an excellent source of vitamin A and natural daylight on the skin provides the best form of vitamin D.

Omega-3-6(9) oil

A good oil with a high omega-3 content ideally should contain GLA (gamma-linoleic acid) as evening primrose or sunflower oil. Oils should always be stored in a cold dark place in glass, never in plastic because they can dissolve traces of fat-soluble toxins.

Brewer's yeast

This is an excellent source of B vitamins and vital minerals such as iron, chromium, copper and zinc. (Ignore the old wives' tales and advice of wacky alternative practitioners that this will cause candida.)

Kelp

This is good for iodine and other minerals for good brain function.

Selenium

This is the only mineral supplement that we recommend. It is an especially good antioxidant to repair oxidative damage to the brain and liver. It is also vital to the immune system, and supplementation with selenium, tryptophan, cysteine and glutamine has been shown to help increase levels of glutathione peroxidase (vital for immune function) which is depleted in some virus infections, especially AIDS, and to relieve some of the symptoms.[72]

FOOD FACTOR 9: DIETARY PRECURSORS OF SOME NEUROTRANSMITTERS

All the known neurotransmitters such as GABA and the monoamine neurotransmitters are manufactured in the brain from precursor substances and are therefore termed non-essential.[73] However, it has been known for some time that the manufacture and release of neurotransmitters depends mainly on the concentration of their precursors in the blood.[74] Ingestion of particular foods can change the physiological functioning of the brain. This produces only subtle effects in healthy individuals but can significantly affect those with depression.

The effect of food is most obvious for the amino acids tryptophan, tyrosine and phenylalanine, the precursors of serotonin, dopamine and noradrenaline respectively. Single meals can influence the brain's uptake of these and modify their conversion to neurotransmitters.[75] The precursors compete for transport into the brain and since there is generally less tryptophan than tyrosine in food, especially high-protein foods, brain levels of tryptophan and the synthesis of serotonin can be blocked by eating too much protein.[76] In contrast, high-carbohydrate meals increase levels of tryptophan and hence serotonin because, although carbohydrates contain little tryptophan, they cause the body to release insulin which locks up competing amino acids in muscle tissue.

Glutamate

Glutamate is normally manufactured in the brain from protein. Together with glycine, it controls an important glutamate receptor, which is important in memory in the brain (Chapter 3). It is also regulated by magnesium and zinc. Glutamate is derived from protein foods such as meat, soya products, nuts, beans and seeds. Interestingly, plant proteins generally contain more glutamate by weight (up to 40 per cent) than animal proteins (11–22 per cent).[77] It is especially rich in tomatoes and some other fruits.

GABA

GABA is synthesised in the brain from glutamic acid with a vitamin B6 derivative as a co-factor. Deficiency in vitamin B6 can result in seizure because of GABA deficiency in the brain. Because of its inhibitory effect on neurons, GABA is also protective during strokes, heart disease or any other event causing a lack of oxygen in the brain.

Serotonin

Serotonin in the brain is synthesised from tryptophan, with iron as a co-factor. It is transported with other amino acids across the blood–brain barrier. The serotonin concentration in the brain is more affected by diet than any other monoamine neurotransmitter, and almost all the tryptophan in the blood is normally converted to serotonin in the brain. Hence diet can be used to improve mental well-being as discussed above. Foods that increase tryptophan in the brain include oats, bananas, avocados, dried dates, red meat, fish, poultry, sesame, chick peas and peanuts.

Perhaps chocolate should be given special mention because it contains alkaloids shown to increase brain serotonin levels. Chocolate also contains phenyl ethylamine, the 'falling in love' chemical, and anandamines, which act like a benign type of cannabis – but beware the caffeine if you suffer from anxiety. The best chocolate is dark and organic; the only sugar this contains is unrefined raw cane sugar.

Dopamine and noradrenaline

L-phenylalanine is a building block for various proteins produced in the body. It can be converted to L-tyrosine, dopamine and noradrenaline. It can be converted (through a separate pathway) to phenylethylamine (PEA) which is a mood enhancer.

Dopamine is synthesised in the brain from tyrosine, its precursor chemical, with iron as a co-factor; vitamin B is also essential for these reactions. Noradrenaline is synthesised from dopamine by an enzyme with oxygen, vitamin C and copper as co-factors. Phenylalanine is high in most protein foods such as red meat, eggs, soya products, nuts (especially almonds and peanuts) and seeds (especially pumpkin seeds) as well as bananas and avocados. Foods that increase levels of tyrosine include soya products, chicken, turkey, fish, peanuts, almonds, avocados, bananas, lima beans, pumpkin and sesame seeds.

Acetylcholine

Acetylcholine is the main neurotransmitter of the peripheral nervous system and is essential for brain function. Low levels are associated with poor learning ability and mental awareness. Choline is its precursor chemical, and occurs as lecithin in many foods such as eggs, soya and peanuts.

FOOD FACTOR 10: HEALTHY DRINKS

Water

It is a good idea to drink lots of water, but it is important to find good sources. Before humankind reached the sort of population densities we have now, especially in cities, and before we began to use large quantities of water for washing cars and manufacturing things, most people would have drunk water from natural sources such as wells, springs or rivers. Unfortunately, the only way of providing adequate water now is to recycle it by treating and reprocessing it at sewage works. We often joke now that when someone in the East End of London drinks a glass of water 15 people have previously drunk the same water.

This water differs significantly from natural water in several ways. First, it lacks the minerals dissolved in many natural waters such as the alkaline elements calcium, magnesium, potassium and lithium which are good for the brain and nervous system. It is also likely to contain tiny traces of water-processing chemicals and disinfection by-products, as well as chemicals from fossil-fuel burning and manufacturing processes and pharmaceutical residues from human and veterinary medicines.

Recycled water potentially creates two main problems – deficiency and toxicity.

Mineral deficiencies

We may not be getting adequate amounts of minerals such as lithium from our drinking water, and this might affect certain people who suffer from bipolar disorder. It is possible that lithium deficiency might cause problems in people whose metabolism is adapted to high levels of lithium, such as occur in the south-west of England or the Mediterranean regions of Europe.[78]

Toxicity

In addition to the neurotoxic actions of chemicals discussed on pages 198–202, pharmaceutical residues in the environment are of increasing concern. A recent survey in the US showed that 38 drinking-water extraction wells contained detectable levels of residues of pharmaceuticals, ranging from hormones and Viagra to chemotherapeutic agents and antidepressants.[79]

Mineral water

Nevertheless we do not recommend mineral water, especially from plastic bottles. Some mineral waters can contain high levels of radioactivity, heavy metals or nitrate, depending on their source. Indeed, some mineral waters would not be legal if they came out of a tap in the UK.

Filtered water

It is far better to filter your tap water and then store it in glass or earthenware in a cool place. We do not recommend elaborate systems of water purification such as reverse osmosis. We prefer systems based on filtration. A simple jug filter is perfectly adequate and this is what we use.

Teas

Green tea is especially good for you because of the powerful antioxidants it contains. Buy it from a Chinese, Japanese or Korean shop and add freshly squeezed lemon, lime or orange juice before drinking for a delicious refreshing cuppa. Herbal teas are generally fine (though you should try to avoid fruit teas that are flavoured with the sort of chemicals used to flavour jellies). Some herbal teas contain herbs known to fight anxiety or depression (see page 127).

Juices and smoothies

Fruit and vegetable juices and smoothies are generally excellent, especially if they are freshly made. We have half a glass of freshly squeezed lemon juice every morning. Smoothies are generally easiest because cleaning up afterwards is so much easier. Simply put all your favourite fruits into a blender and process to produce drinks that are packed with vitamins and other powerful antioxidants. Avoid commercial juice drinks though, which can be full of white sugar and other additives, and smoothies containing yoghurt or other dairy produce. Many colas and squashes can also be packed with additives, including tartrazine in yellow- or orange-coloured drinks. Avoid all diet drinks that contain aspartame or other man-made 'sugars'.

The problem with caffeine

Caffeine in coffee or strong tea should be avoided by those with anxiety. It blocks receptors that normally inhibit glutamate release and inhibits the effect of GABA on receptors, which also increases anxiety in vulnerable people. Coffee's effect takes hold within about 20 minutes and lasts for two to three hours. Tea has a weaker, longer-lasting effect because it contains less caffeine and its caffeine is in a form which is released more slowly. Drinking too much strong tea or coffee can cause vitamin B1 deficiency which can lead to generalised anxiety. Jane never drinks coffee because she knows that it will make her feel agitated in seconds.

Drinking chocolate also contains caffeine, but chocolate also contains lots of feel-good chemicals and nutrients too. Drink it in moderation made with soya milk rather than dairy.

Alcohol – the importance of moderation

Alcohol in moderation is fine for most people and it can appear to help with anxiety in the short term, but in some circumstances it can make matters much worse. It initially raises levels of neurotransmitters, but they are then excreted from the body making people feel low. Wine can also contain additives such as sodium sulphite that make some people particularly ill. We enjoy organic beer or cider. An occasional single malt whisky or gin and tonic (not diet) is also fine, but never have alcohol if you are depressed. It will surely make matters worse.

CASE HISTORY: *John*

John was in his early sixties, a retired insurance broker who had a very successful career. After a couple of years of retirement his wife, Sue, noticed that he was becoming increasingly angry and aggressive between periods of being totally withdrawn. He was eventually persuaded to see his doctor, who referred him to a geriatric psychiatrist. John was reluctant to go and refused to have a brain scan or any other diagnostic test. His wife was extremely upset but agreed to try to improve his diet. Since he never cooked, this was something she could control. John had typically eaten a rich diet dominated by animal foods, especially meat and cheese, with very little in the way of fruit or vegetables and he also drank quite a lot of wine. Sue removed all the cheese and other dairy products, which are a source of brain-damaging calcium ions and saturated fats from his diet and bought game rather than farmed meat. He was also persuaded to limit eggs to one or two a week. He was given lots of vegetables and salads and persuaded to have fruits, mainly as smoothies. He also took the food supplements recommended on pp 238. After about six weeks, his wife noticed that his memory had improved significantly and he appeared more settled and patient. Six months on, she feels he has made a dramatic recovery from a diagnosis of major depression, which she confessed she had feared was the onset of Alzheimer's disease.

CASE HISTORY: *Maggie*

Maggie was the wife of a headmaster in a pleasant, rural area. Her husband was always smiling and happy and was well-liked by all the community. Maggie had two sons but was painfully thin and suffered serious bouts of depression, which failed to respond to medication or ECT. She and her husband were persuaded to improve her diet, which basically relied on cheese and apple sandwiches which she had used to control her food intake when she began to suffer from anorexia in her teens. She was persuaded to follow the Plant Programme of eating, and although she will never be the extrovert that her husband is, she certainly feels and copes much better with her family and increasingly supports her husband's career.

Chapter Eleven

The Wrong End of the Telescope

THE TWENTIETH CENTURY HAS seen great strides in socio-economic development throughout the West, with a vast improvement in material standards of living, but we appear as a society to have paid a high price in terms of deteriorating mental health. The advancement in levels of education and access to health and social services that has helped to overcome many infectious illnesses, mainly by better public health such as improved sanitation, food preparation and personal hygiene, has been accompanied by a dramatic rise in many other diseases, especially anxiety and depression.

The facts are stark and shocking. In Britain today a staggering one person in six will suffer from depression or a chronic anxiety disorder at some time in their lives.[1] In the US a mental disorder will affect one in five people during their lifetimes; and people born after the Second World War are twice as likely to develop a mental illness as their parents.[2] These dry statistics understate the severity of the situation, because mental illness affects not only the lives of sufferers but also of their partners, families and friends. This means that in Britain one family in three is likely to be affected at some point.[2]

The human misery involved is incalculable. Lewis Wolpert, the distinguished biologist, writes that his own depression was the worst experience of his life.[3] He goes on to say: 'It was not just feeling very low, depressed in the commonly used sense of the word. I was in a state that bears no resemblance to anything I had experienced before. I was seriously ill. I was totally self-involved, negative and thought about suicide most of the time.'

Indeed, it has been suggested that in Britain today chronic anxiety and crippling depression are the biggest causes of misery, far outweighing poverty as a cause of social deprivation.[4]

Depression is one of the most serious health threats worldwide, with more working days lost to it than any other illness, and it is predicted to increase further so that by 2020 it may become the second greatest cause of premature death and disability (after cardiovascular disease) worldwide. In the world as a whole almost a million people take their own lives every year, more than the number murdered or killed in war. Almost all people who kill themselves have some form of mental illness, often combined with substance abuse from attempts at self-medication.

Post-natal depression, which is at the heart of Janet's story, is particularly important, partly because it is so common and partly because it occurs at such a critical time in the lives of the mother, her baby and her family. A UK Inquiry into Maternal Deaths reports that psychiatric disorders contributed to 12 per cent of all perinatal deaths.[5] Suicide is a leading cause of perinatal death in the UK, second only to cardiovascular disease.[6]

As well as the appalling human misery involved, these illnesses are hugely expensive. In Britain about 40 per cent of all disability, as reflected by people on incapacity benefits, is due to mental illness.[7] This is overwhelmingly due to anxiety disorders and depression. In the UK, the total loss of output due to depression and chronic anxiety is estimated at £12 billion a year.[7] This includes £11 billion paid to people diagnosed with depression, £276 million to sufferers of anxiety disorders and £122 million to those suffering from severe stress.[8] In the US mental disorders cost more than $150 billion annually, about $67 billion of which is for direct health costs, including medication, the rest being for social services, disability benefits and lost productivity. Nearly 75 per cent of those affected will have had at least one episode by the time they are 21 years old. Untreated, people with serious conditions such as major depression and OCD can face a lifetime of disability, with all the individual problems this creates, as well as the loss to the economy of the contribution that sufferers could make if they were well.

Mental illness can be the cause of isolation, and even stigma, for the sufferers. It tends to be treated sensationally as a focus of fear by the media, or as something to be swept under the carpet and ignored by society. Although charities such as Mind, SANE and the Samaritans campaign for better treatment of mental illness, they have so far had much less success in changing public perceptions and media attitudes than the cancer charities, particularly those for breast cancer. Consequently, there has been little or no public pressure for improved treatment. In an article in the *Evening Standard* on 20 August 2007 the mental health services in the UK were said to be being 'bled of resources', with widening gaps in services. Mental health was said to be the Cinderella service of the NHS, with primary care trusts 'borrowing' money from this area all the time to plug holes in their budgets. This was confirmed by a recent survey by the Sainsbury Centre for Mental Health that found that more than half of England's mental-health trusts have seen money diverted away from them to pay for deficits in other local health services. This was thought to reflect the fact that mental-health patients are less pushy than other patients.[9] Both articles also made the point that, with a few exceptions, no one is speaking out about the cuts. While politicians boast of their efforts to improve cancer treatment and use it as a performance indicator for our health services, the politics of mental health appear almost entirely focused on the control of the sick. Let us briefly consider the difference in the way that physical and emotional pain is typically treated by health-care systems.

PHYSICAL VERSUS EMOTIONAL PAIN

Imagine that you are in severe physical pain, say in the area of your abdomen, and you go to see your doctor. You tell them about your pain and they spend about five minutes listening to you before reaching for the prescription pad. You take the pills prescribed which have unpleasant side effects but after a few weeks the pain is no better and you return to talk to your doctor. When you tell them about the pain they simply increase the dose and your side effects get worse but the pain does not improve. You return to see your doctor who simply changes the pills but the new pills don't work either and you are forced to return to your doctor; and this goes on for weeks and all the time your pain is becoming more intense. Eventually you are sent to see a specialist. You are given an hour of their time but at the end you are simply given more pills. Imagine that the situation begins to deteriorate further and you are now offered electrical therapy, which effectively passes an electric current through the organ deemed to be causing the pain, a method for which there is little or no evidence that it works but which can have serious side effects. All this misery, and at no time have any tests been carried out to determine precisely what is wrong with your abdomen.

If cancer patients were treated in this way there would be outrage, and yet this is precisely what happens to many people with anxiety and depression when they turn to their health professionals for help with their intense emotional pain.

DRUGS WITHOUT DIAGNOSIS

One of the main problems is that we continue to put too many resources into a system based simply on using pills alone to suppress symptoms. Medication remains the treatment of choice for anxiety and depression by most doctors and psychiatrists. In the last ten years, consumption of antidepressants has doubled in most advanced Western countries.[10] Today more than 11 million people in the US and more than 2 million people in the UK are taking them. Antidepressants are among the top selling drugs in the US, with about one in eight Americans estimated to have taken them, half of them for more than a year.[10] In the year 2000, over 20 million prescriptions were written for antidepressants in England alone, at a cost of £296 million.[10] One view is that doctors and psychiatrists, influenced by pharmaceutical-industry marketing, are prescribing antidepressants for people who are experiencing normal emotional reactions, such as sadness, in response to adverse life experiences. Professor Rapley,

Professor of Clinical Psychology at the University of East London, is quoted as saying, 'What I object to is the intellectual trickery and how the drugs industry has made us believe that when we feel sad we have something fundamentally wrong with us that needs correcting.'[11]

A review of the effectiveness of SSRI antidepressants in the *New Scientist* in 2005 found that there is no evidence that they make people less depressed; they are not helping people return to work, nor are they preventing or reducing suicide.[12] The authors of this review concluded that such antidepressants prevent people tackling the underlying causes of their depression and are no better than placebos (dummy pills).

Indeed, all treatments for depression need to be assessed against the high recovery rate of patients who receive no treatment at all. Suicide attempts in the Netherlands have increased during a time when antidepressant use has also increased.[13] Psychiatrist Joanna Moncrieff also believes that medicalising people's distress only compounds their problems and is not backed up by evidence.[14]

Charles Medawar and Andrew Herxheimer have studied the side effects of the antidepressant Seroxat (paroxetine) using the yellow-card system, which is used in the UK to report the side effects of prescription drugs. The system, which they describe as 'chaotic and misconceived', recently underestimated suspicions of suicide and there was no evidence of regulatory follow-up of reports of suicidal behaviour and injury/poisoning. Medawar was also the first to conclude that the risk of withdrawal symptoms from SSRIs is about 25 per cent. For about 15 years the regulator had failed to report this problem.[15]

The problem of the overuse of pills is made worse by a lack of proper diagnosis. Outside the best private clinics, the diagnosis and treatment of anxiety and depression are still based mainly on an empirical or 'suck it and see' approach, so the wrong drugs may be being prescribed.

THE THINKING OF THE CUCKOO'S NEST

So what are we doing about this dire situation? The answer is 'certainly nothing effective!' Indeed, most effort on behalf of the government is still about controlling those who are seriously mentally ill. The thinking is still that of the cuckoo's nest.

In the UK the existing Mental Health Act dates from 1983. Although this act was an improvement on previous acts (for example, homosexuality is explicitly excluded from being considered as a mental illness) it nevertheless focuses on controlling the mentally ill and compelling them to accept treatment and, in some cases, incarceration. A new act now going through its committee stages in Parliament shows the same underlying philosophy. At its best, such legislation fails to improve the situation and at its worst, it drives people who are mentally ill away from help for fear of what could happen to them.

THE WRONG END OF THE TELESCOPE

We believe that politicians and society in general are looking at the problem of mental health through the wrong end of the telescope. They continue to focus on controlling the sick, when they should instead be focusing on the healthcare system which has stumbled on, almost unchanged, for decades. It is a system that relies on pills and potions and primitive Victorian methods of treatment such as ECT and which is staffed by health professionals many of whom know little or nothing about the organ they are supposed to be treating. It is this shambling state of affairs that needs urgent attention.

The human brain is the most complex system in the known universe and yet we continue to allow people who may know little or nothing about it to prescribe medication, and indeed in some cases to compel people to take it – or subject it to electrical shocks. We would not believe it credible if computers were treated in this way and yet this is how we treat the brain, which is far more complex than any computer.

The mentally ill do not want to be ill. Neither of us knows of any worse misery, including for the friends and families of sufferers, so what needs to be done about the system? What can be achieved by legislation?

Education and training of specialists in mental illness

When Jane went with her younger son to discuss his wish to follow a career in medicine with the careers advisor, an experienced teacher at his school, she was taken aback by the teacher's response. Instead of saying 'Wonderful! How can we help you?' he said, 'Oh what a shame; Tom is far too good a scientist to go into medicine.' When pressed, the teacher explained that for a medical career the school normally took pupils who were good at biology and gave them lots of help to achieve the grades needed in chemistry and physics, even if they were not particularly good at these subjects. They were, he said, unlikely to need much in-depth understanding of these subjects in their medical training. This is fine for surgeons, radiographers and even GPs, but it is not acceptable for doctors who are destined to work on treating the mentally ill using invasive chemical or physical approaches.

Psychiatry, science and historical abuses of human rights

What emerges from reviewing much of the treatment of the mentally ill is the apparent lack of any scientific basis. It strikes Jane as odd, for example, that it took psychiatrists about 70 years longer to realise that electrical flow could be generated in a conductor (the human brain) using a changing magnetic field than Earth scientists, who began to use the method from the 1930s to induce electrical flow to explore for conductive sulphide ore deposits.[16] Why did psychiatrists keep using the much cruder method of ECT to pass an electrical current through the brain when they could have induced the brain to do this using magnetic induction? Because they did not know enough basic physics?

It also strikes Jane as odd that standard techniques of determining levels of organic chemicals such as GCMS and HPLC are not used in diagnosis before drugs are prescribed. Even the terminology in mental health is confused and confusing. For example, most scientists and engineers use stress to mean the force or pressure applied and strain to indicate the resulting effects on the metal or substance being subjected to stress. Medicine uses stress to mean both stress and strain.

In the past, psychiatry has used methods that must be of concern to all civilised people. Frontal lobotomy, at the height of its popularity in the 1940s and 1950s, particularly in the US, was promoted by some of the most enthusiastic proponents of the procedure as a way of controlling large numbers of those considered to be society's worst misfits, including communists and homosexuals. In the past, little attention was paid to what happened to those subjected to lobotomies after treatment. Rose Kennedy, President John F. Kennedy's temperamental sister, underwent the operation at the age of 23 and spent the next 60 years of her life in a mental institution. Frances Farmer, the rebellious Hollywood actress and political activist, whose outspoken behaviour was also 'cured' by a lobotomy, rapidly declined and ended her days as a hotel clerk.

Many of those who underwent such surgery were rendered unable to speak for themselves and those subjected to the cruder forms of surgery are no longer alive. One survivor's recollections were published in the *Sunday Times* as 'a rare testimony of someone still lucid and intensely angry about his brain surgery, particularly as the family consent came from his mother, an alcoholic, when she was drunk'. He is quoted as saying, 'My mother thought doctors were Gods.'[17]

The use of ECT grew out of a late-Victorian fascination with electricity, and although it has been used in the West since the 1930s there is still no rational scientific understanding of how such a treatment could work and there are serious concerns about its use. On 26 October 2006 an article in the (Irish) *Sunday Independent,* headed '"Inhumane" shock therapy is on rise', quoted consultant psychiatrist Dr Michael Corry as likening the procedure to 'something you would see in death camps ... The bottom line is it causes brain damage. It's barbaric. We're talking about a human rights issue here.' A patient treated with ECT is quoted as saying, 'I think patients are saying yes because they are so gullible and because they think doctors would never do anything that could harm them. I definitely think people are going to start suing.' The article concludes with the results of a survey carried out by the UK mental health charity Mind that found that 84 per cent of respondents had suffered side effects from ECT, including permanent memory loss and the inability to read, write and concentrate, as well as headaches and confusion.

In the 1940s and 1950s, the extensive use of ECT in frequent high doses for long periods of time produced harmful effects in patients and there is also evidence that it was used to control behaviour in mental institutions. Nearly 40 per cent of patients suffered complications and the overall death rate was one in 1,000. ECT was administered without anaesthesia and bone fractures caused by muscle spasms under treatment were a serious problem. There were also claims that ECT caused permanent brain damage.[18]

PSYCHIATRISTS AS SCIENTISTS

Beginning with Freud, psychiatrists who are also neurologists and neuroscientists have made major contributions to the science of mental illness. Joseph Schiildkraut, for example, in his classic paper 'The Catecholamine Hypothesis of Affective Disorders', published in *The American Journal of Psychiatry* in 1965, showed that many mental disorders are related to chemical imbalances in the brain. Helen Mayberg, who has developed the system for implanting pacemaker-like electrodes in specific parts of the brain to treat depression, and David Servan-Schreiber who has pioneered non-invasive methods of healing the emotional brain via the body, are neurologists or neuroscientists respectively as well as psychiatrists. They have made enormous contributions to developing effective and humane methods of treating mental illness based on sound science. Daniel Amen, who has pioneered the use of diagnostic brain scans, despite the roars of disapproval from the dinosaurs of the psychiatric industry, is also such a doctor. Unfortunately, they are the exceptions.

ROCKET SCIENCE

Many psychiatrists have only a poor or superficial knowledge of the brain. In Daniel Amen's words: 'They are the only medical specialists who rarely look at the organ they treat. They will prescribe medication, psychotherapy, ECT or a host of other treatments that will change brain function but will not know which areas of the patient's brain work too hard and which do not work hard enough.'[19]

A similar point is made by Nobel prizewinning neuroscientist Eric Kandel, who has said that it is time to transform the healing art of psychiatry into a modern discipline. Psychiatry's ageing interpretative framework, he argues, must be reworked to incorporate our new understanding of the biological bases of memory and emotion.[20]

Many psychiatrists appear to know even less of the physiology and chemistry of the brain. The problem is summed up by Lechin, in relation to medicine in general, as follows: 'The practice of medicine is divided into two camps of doctors: scientists and clinicians. The former acquire knowledge about physiology, pathophysiology, pharmacology, neurochemistry, neuroendocrinology, immunology, genetics, biochemistry and many other disciplines. Unfortunately these scientific doctors do not practise medicine. Conversely, many clinical practitioners possess only superficial knowledge of these disciplines and so are limited to rudimentary and simplistic diagnostic and therapeutic procedures for suppressing symptoms. Such doctors spend most of their working life acquiring skills and perfecting techniques and so are unable to keep abreast of scientific advances.'[21]

He goes on to say, 'Science should make an incursion into the practice of medicine. While doctors are trained as technicians, the pharmaceutical industry prescribes treatments to patients.' This is surely true of most psychiatrists. How can such specialists be allowed to continue to use invasive psychoactive drug treatments and physical methods such as ECT and psychosurgery?

General psychiatrists prescribing powerful drugs or worse still treatments such as ECT based on simple case-history information was bad enough in the 1940s and 1950s, but it is surely unacceptable now. Can anyone imagine having invasive treatment for a heart problem on such a basis?

Interestingly, Helen Mayberg, the distinguished neurologist who now has 'psychiatrist' in her title, finds this quite strange, 'considering I rejected psychiatry as too nebulous a discipline. I didn't like the tool kit,' she explains.[22]

Psychiatry is often a Cinderella subject, looked down on by other medical professionals. Psychiatrists are often referred to by names such as 'trick cyclists' or 'shrinks', reflecting the lack of a firm scientific basis for the discipline. On the other hand we often use the term 'brain surgeon' to indicate someone who is the epitomy of cleverness, who would understand rocket science because they understand the workings of the most complex object in the known universe, the human brain. We need specialists working with the mentally ill who are not only capable of understanding rocket science but are able to advance it in relation to the brain. Psychiatrists should not be mediocre doctors who were good at descriptive biology at school and saw psychiatry as a fast track to becoming a consultant.

At the beginning of the twenty-first century it is surely time to ensure that invasive physical treatments for mental illness can be prescribed and administered only by specialists who have an in-depth knowledge of the brain and nervous system and its workings. Interestingly, the most science-based methods of treating serious mental illness such as DBS now involve brain surgeons, not psychiatrists. Nevertheless, some people are still treated with ECT and even psychosurgery by psychiatrists without any proper diagnosis being made first. We also need to train specialists in interpreting functional brain scans for the diagnosis of mental illness, just as we use specialist radiographers to interpret sophisticated scans used in the diagnosis and treatment of cancer or heart disease.

Drugs have produced major advances in the treatment of mental illness, but their value is diminished and much suffering caused by the lack of proper targeting. Great strides could be made if the improved methods of diagnosis used in private clinics were made more widely available. GPs should be more aware of them and trained in their use.

Much effort needs to be devoted to developing and standardising diagnostic techniques for mental illness, to bring them to the same standards as those used for physical illnesses. Indeed, more work needs to be done generally in standardising terminology – between the Amen and Lechin schools, for example. The conditions being treated need to be related to problems with brain function rather than being diagnosed on the basis of overlapping symptoms and subjective case histories. New functional brain-scanning systems should be developed, adopted and standardised, and all psychiatrists should be trained in their use – and in neuroscience generally.

The best private clinics in the US use techniques such as functional brain imaging to diagnose their patients' illnesses and to monitor their progress. Treatment involves a holistic approach that includes not only medication but also nutritional programmes, exercise and social and emotional support. This is a far cry from the treatment most people with anxiety or depression experience using public healthcare systems such as that in the UK.

All specialists who treat mental disorders such as anxiety and depression, including psychiatric consultants, should be required to pass advanced examinations in the neurology, physiology and biochemistry of the brain and nervous system. Such specialists should be designated neurophysicians to indicate that they are qualified to work on the human brain and they should replace psychiatrists. This is where legislation should be directed first and as a matter of urgency.

BETTER-TRAINED GPS AND NURSES

We believe that the new Mental Health Act should address incentives to ensure that doctors and nurses in primary care adopt best practice in treating patients with stress, anxiety and depression. This should involve appropriate talking therapy and guidance on nutritional and lifestyle factors, as well as properly targeted medication based on sound diagnosis. Ideally, some doctors and nurses working in primary care practices should have qualifications in mental health and this should involve training in the workings of the brain and nervous system.

General physicians or practitioners (GPs in the UK) do need better training in helping to prevent and treat mental illness, including helping their patients to deal with stress. (Studies suggest that as many as 75 per cent of visits to GPs in the UK are related to stress.)[23] Doctors need to know when to recommend counselling and other methods of healing the mind before considering medication. Recently the UK government has increased spending on cognitive behavioural therapy (CBT) but much more use should be made of counsellors to help people cope with their real-life problems rather than prescribing medication. Someone whose husband has just died or left her for another woman needs help in coming to terms with her new situation – not pills.

Doctors should provide good nutritional advice, and senior practice nurses should be trained to help patients to make lifestyle changes such as incorporating good nutrition and exercise into their daily routine. There is now much credible scientific evidence, including evidence from medical trials, that nutrition is the key to treating many mental illnesses, including serious conditions such as bipolar disorder. Professor Basant Puri, in the Imaging Sciences Department, Hammersmith Hospital, part of Imperial College, London has produced compelling evidence that the fat profile of the diet is crucial for mental health, including that of children.[24] We should be eating foods high in essential fatty acids and cutting down dramatically on trans fats and saturated fats. Most nurses and doctors appear to be totally ignorant of such findings and they continue to push dairy produce, including cheese, despite it being officially designated as junk food by the UK Food Standards Agency because of the levels of saturated fat and salt it contains. This is also despite the fact that dairy contains staggeringly high levels of calcium, which have been shown by other studies to cause tissue damage to the brain associated with Parkinson's and dementia.[25] They need to ensure that all their advice, not just their advice on medication, is evidence based.

GPs should be trained never to prescribe pills for anxiety and depression without a proper diagnosis of what is wrong with their patients. We can think of no other serious illness for which diagnostic tests are not carried out before prescribing. (Quite the reverse, in fact: for many other illnesses, doctors frequently resort to tests in preference to using their professional experience and judgement to make a diagnosis.)

OTHER HEALTH PROFESSIONALS

There is overwhelming evidence that psychological therapies such as cognitive behavioural therapy (CBT) or psychodynamic counselling (PDC) can lift at least half of those affected out of their depression or chronic anxiety and that the official guidelines from the National Institute for Health and Clinical Excellence for England and Wales (NICE) state that 'psychological treatments should be available to all people with depression or anxiety disorders or schizophrenia, unless the problem is very mild or recent'.[26] Such therapy is as effective as drugs in the short term and has more long-lasting effects than drugs in the longer term. Indeed in the case of anxiety people are unlikely to relapse after therapy.

Although the government has recently made available an extra £170 million for CBT, the NICE guidelines cannot be implemented fully because we have far too few therapists so that all that can be offered in most cases is medication. This vicious circle that causes such misery and suffering to millions will be broken only with a massive switch of resources. 'The Depression Report: A New Deal for Depression and Anxiety Disorders', prepared by the LSE, calculates that the cost of psychological therapies would be £750 per patient, which would be paid for if they returned to work for just one month. Put another way, it would cost the economy just £0.6 billion rather than the massive £21 billion that depression and anxiety disorders presently cost the economy.[26]

BRINGING IN MORE COMMON SENSE

Social workers are often involved in helping mentally ill people. All too often, poor decisions about their care are reported in the media and this becomes particularly emotive in situations where small children are involved. Only recently the UK press has reported at length on the horrific murder of two small children by their schizophrenic mother. Such reports do little to improve sympathy for mentally ill people and many of us feel a sense of unease as we hear yet another bureaucratic justification from some director of social services or other wheeled out to explain what has gone wrong. Many social workers on the front line are young and with academic rather than real-life qualifications and are often working under considerable pressure.

We would propose putting the seriously mentally ill capable of living in the community in the day-to-day care of social services, under the direction of magistrates or their equivalent. The involvement of older people, some of whom have raised their own families successfully and are known to be worldly wise, would do a great deal to improve decision-making about the social care of the mentally ill. Such a system would be more cost effective than the present one and would be seen as bringing in common sense.

PSYCHIATRIC WARDS AND MENTAL INSTITUTIONS

For in-patients the outlook is often particularly poor. Once again the problem is too great a reliance on drugs and treatments such as ECT to treat the mentally ill. We know many people who are very worried about loved ones apparently left heavily drugged to languish in unpleasant psychiatric wards. We recently visited a psychiatric ward in a wealthy borough in south-east England where the staff just watched their patients through two-way mirrors and spent no time talking to or comforting their patients. The ward was a mixed ward in every sense, with males and females and psychotic and non-psychotic patients left with nothing to do but watch the television or play computer games. The only beneficial thing we found was a snooker table, but this appeared to be little used. The library was permanently locked and there was no 'green space' for the patients to get fresh air or exercise.

It is interesting that many aspects of the old asylums combined methods now shown scientifically to help restore the mind and spirit. The standard of care varied markedly, but the best were in garden settings where simple nutritious meals were provided and there were daily routines involving exercise and meditation. Physical work was encouraged and some had farms that helped in-patients reconnect with nature as well as growing food. An almost universally accepted criticism of the closure of old-fashioned asylums is the loss of gardens and access to green space for patients. Some gardening projects run by hospitals for the mentally ill are being reintroduced. They are often aimed at transforming derelict areas into havens for wildlife, thereby promoting social inclusion and employability as well as patients' mental well-being in the community. There should be much more emphasis on ecotherapy centres.

Much more needs to be done to help treat in-patients effectively while making life bearable for the small number of people who must be detained for their own safety or that of others. There should be a return to some of the best aspects of the old asylums, especially the nourishing food, meaningful work and a routine involving exercise and relaxation. There should certainly be single-sex wards, and ideally patients who are dangerously psychotic should be treated separately from people suffering from mood disorders for whom stress reduction is essential.

THE MEDICAL PROFESSION AND THE PREVENTION OF ANXIETY AND DEPRESSION

In common with its approach to many other diseases, Western medicine generally treats mental illness by treating the symptoms after they have appeared, with little or no attention directed to fundamental causes and prevention. As we discussed above, anxiety and depression are becoming more and more common and costly in the human misery and deprivation they cause, as well as in the direct costs involved to the economy. In environmental sciences, concentrating on the treatment of symptoms is now regarded as an old-fashioned 'end of pipe' solution. As long ago as the 1970s, it was recognised that it was far better to look at the full life cycle of a process, for example in a factory, and to minimise environmental impacts at each stage rather than wait to deal with some unpleasant effluent at the end. We think that it would be far better to view mental illness in a similar way, with much greater emphasis on prevention.

Unfortunately, the evidence from the UK, at least, is that doctors who care about public health in relation to mental health are the exception.

There are, of course, enlightened doctors who take an interest in public policy and public health, like Dr Richard Jackson in the US and Dr Stephen Holgate, a member of the Royal Commission on Environmental Pollution in the UK. Such doctors clearly see patients as people not 'interesting cases of ...', and take a world view of health problems. They make an important contribution to public health, especially mental health, by influencing policy. Their input is needed, for example, in housing and planning policy to ensure that we develop sustainable communities with access to green space for recreation and walking rather than soulless estates that are designed for cars and are particularly bad for children and the elderly. We also need more doctors who fight for good nutrition and tell the government if our diet is lacking key nutrients such as omega-3 fatty acids or zinc or lithium, and doctors prepared to say if too many neurotoxic chemicals are being sprayed around as pesticides, for example. We also need such doctors to be involved in the design of education systems, to help young people to achieve their potential without damaging their mental health. We propose a new medical specialty of mental health consultant in public health.

Healing society's anxiety and depression

We believe that there is now so much excellent reproducible science on the causes of mood disorders that we have a strong evidence base with which to prevent and treat stress, anxiety and depression in individuals and society in general. We hope that by reading this book you are better equipped to help yourself and those you love and care for.

INTO A NEW DAY

However ill you are now, try to remember that we both felt, in the depth of our despair, that we would always be ill and that there was nothing anybody could do to help us. We are both quite well and happy now. We both think we benefited from our experiences and that we are now better people and better able to understand and help others. In the words of the Chinese poem to an ugly slave, written in the twelfth century by Xin Qiji: 'Now having known all the taste of sorrow we simply say "it is a good day, it is a fine autumn morning".'

Twelve Golden Guidelines for Those Whose Lives are Affected by Anxiety or Depression

As we have learned in this book, there is much that can be done to help prevent and treat anxiety and depression. Here we give you 12 golden guidelines to help you.

We offer some suggestions ranging from avoiding stress in your day-to-day life to increasing self-esteem and competences. We also suggest that if you are already a sufferer you should use a holistic approach to treatment, involving some of the following: medication based on accurate and meaningful diagnosis, appropriate talking therapies, acupuncture or other methods of communicating with the unconscious mind, exercise and, importantly, good nutrition.

1 Finding appropriate help

Serious stress is undoubtedly a key factor leading to anxiety and depression. The major factors that cause individuals to become stressed differ and may be related to childhood events locked away in the implicit memory. If something happens later in life that resonates with such memories, unpleasant feelings can be triggered, precipitating mental illness. Try to find a therapist who will help you identify the factors that precipitate your illness and help you to develop coping strategies. Keep a diary to record situations that cause you stress and work on eliminating such situations or reducing their impact on you. If you know you are vulnerable to anxiety or depression try to find counselling to help you come to terms with serious losses and setbacks.

2 Day-to-day stresses

Background levels of stress caused by factors such as uncomfortable shoes or clothes, being on strict diets, or following the wrong daily routine can add to your overall burden of stress and make you more vulnerable to anxiety and depression. Follow the advice in Chapter 9. Note the things that irritate you and work on reducing their impact. If you have worries about practical problems such as money, enlist the help of the Citizens' Advice Bureau. It is free.

3 Drugs and alcohol

Never self-medicate with alcohol or recreational drugs, however stressed you feel, and never try to keep going on caffeine when you feel under pressure. These substances can actually precipitate mental illness if you abuse them.

4 Balance

Try to ensure that your life is balanced. If you spend all your time working to achieve career or professional goals try to find more time for friends and family. Above all, try to find time for you, to go for a walk in an attractive park or garden or pursue a hobby or sport that you enjoy, or just go for tea and a chat with friends. Going for a picnic costs next to nothing. If you are a workaholic, as Jane used to be, this is something you need to recognise and then move into your new way of life gradually but purposefully. If, on the other hand, you are always tired, depressed and lethargic, slouched in a darkened room watching the television, you need to introduce more activity into your life, especially physical activity. Again, do this gradually in a way that you can sustain. Start with a short walk in the most attractive green space you can find and build up gradually, remembering to praise yourself for your achievements.

5 Recharging your batteries

Try to ensure that, in addition to some daily physical exercise, you also have a period of relaxation every day. Have at least one day a week when you can 'switch off' completely. Stay with friends for a weekend occasionally to help put things in a different perspective. Try to ensure that you have adequate restorative sleep.

6 Relationships and isolation

Strong harmonious relationships are essential for the emotional brain. Try to improve your relationships at all levels, with your partner, family and friends by thinking of their needs as well as your own. If you feel isolated socially, try to join a group. Think carefully about the type of things you enjoy and then go to your local library and ask for information on local activities. Going to church can be a good way of connecting with your local community. It is also a way of giving yourself a mental work out by going over all the things you regret, especially in your relations with others, and affirming your intention to do better in the future. Science shows that, whatever the illness, those who have belief in God do better.

7 Materialism

Try to invest in interests rather than things. Spend money on eating with family and friends, going to the cinema or theatre or having aromatherapy or reiki sessions rather than buying yet more things to worry about.

8 Food

Try to eat good food and eliminate junk and convenience food from your life. Follow the dietary advice in Chapter 10 and in the book *Eating for Better Health,* which includes lots of recipes that are practical, nutritious and good for physical and mental well-being.[1] Preparing and cooking good food with others is beneficial for everyone.

9 Man-made chemicals

Try to eliminate as many man-made chemicals from your life as possible by following the advice in Chapter 9.

10 Self-esteem

Improve your self-esteem by working on your appearance, but don't take this to extremes. It is important to work on people skills, such as conversation and listening, too. And don't forget to smile!

11 Anxiety and depression

If the worst comes to the worst and you become anxious or depressed, seek the help of your doctor but try to get help with counselling and other types of therapy rather than simply popping pills without a proper diagnosis. Talking therapies are particularly effective in treating anxiety, for which relapse is unlikely. Don't despair, and remember that most cases of depression resolve themselves. Try to be patient and don't give up hope.

If you are seriously depressed and you are advised to take drugs, ask that a urine sample be analysed to determine which of your neurotransmitters are affected, before you take prescription drugs. There are different types of depression, and the wrong drug could make matters worse. If you are referred to a psychiatrist, try to ensure that it is someone trained in neuroscience who uses methods such as functional brain scans for diagnosis rather than a simple case history.

12 Helping others

Finally, when you recover try to remember to help others especially those with anxiety or depressive illnesses. They are not infectious diseases and helping others can be very beneficial and rewarding. Having been a sufferer yourself you will more fully understand.

Notes

Introduction

1 Amen, D.G., *Neuropsychiatry*, Vol 2(1) (2001),

www.neuropsychiatryreviews.com/feb01/npt_feb01_spect.html

2 Jane Plant, *Your Life in Your Hands: Understand, Prevent and Overcome Breast Cancer and Ovarian Cancer*, 4th edition, Virgin Books (2007).

3 Jane Plant and Gill Tidey, *Understanding, Preventing and Overcoming Osteoporosis*, Virgin Books (2003).

4 Jane Plant, *Prostate Cancer: Understand, Prevent and Overcome*, 2nd edition, Virgin Books (2007).

Chapter 1

1 Katharina Dalton and Wendy Holton, *Depression after Childbirth: How to Recognize, Treat, and Prevent Postnatal Depression*, 4th edition, Oxford University Press (2001).

Chapter 2

1 Allan V. Horwitz and Jerome C. Wakefield, *Loss of Sorrow: How psychiatry transformed normal sorrow into depressive disorder*, Oxford University Press (2007).

2 The Centre for Economic Performance's Mental Health Policy Group, *The Depression Report*. The London School of Economics and Political Science (2006).

3 Rakel, R.E., *Textbook of family practice*, 6th edition, W.B. Saunders (2005), pp. 115–24; APA Task force, 'Schizophrenia and other diagnostic disorders' in *Diagnostic and statistical manual of mental disorders*, 4th edition (DSM–iv), American Psychiatric Association (1994), pp. 273–315.

4 www.4therapy.com/consumer/life_topics/category/110 /sadness&%3B+depression

5 *The Depression Report: A New Deal for Depression and Anxiety Disorders*. A

report by The Centre for Economic Performance's Mental Health Policy Group, The London School of Economics & Political Science. *Observer* (18 June 2006).

6 'Stress-related and psychological disorders', www.hse.gov.uk/statistics/causdis/stress.htm

7 'Psychosocial Working conditions in Britain', Health and Safety Executive (2007).

8 Nixon, P., 'Hyperventilation and cardiac symptoms', *Internal Medicine*, 10(12) (1989), pp. 67–84.

9 Beales, D., 'Beyond mind-body dualism: implications for patient care', *Journal of Holistic Healthcare*, 1(3) (2004), pp. 15–22.

10 Herbert, J., et al, 'Do corticosteroids damage the brain?' *Journal of Neuroendocrinology*, Vol 18 (2006), pp. 393–411.

11 *The Depression Report: A New Deal for Depression and Anxiety Disorders*. A report by The Centre for Economic Performance's Mental Health Policy Group, The London School of Economics & Political Science. *Observer* (18 June 2006).

12 www.nhsdirect.nhs.uk

13 Clark, D.M., 'A cognitive approach to panic', *Behaviour Research and Therapy*, 24 (1986), pp. 461–72; Treatment of panic disorder. *NIH Consens Statement* 9(2) (1991), pp. 1–24.

14 Crazier, W.R. and Alden, L.E., *International Handbook of Social Anxiety*, Wiley (2001).

15 Magee, W.J., et al, 'Agoraphobia, simple phobia, and social phobia in the National Comorbidity Survey', *Archives of General Psychiatry*, 53 (1996), pp. 159–68.

16 Clark, D.M. and Wells, A., 'A cognitive model of social phobias', In Heinberg, R.G. and others. *Social Phobia: Diagnosis, Assessment and Treatment*, Guilford Press (1995).

17 *The Times* (26 November 2007).

18 Claire Ainsworth, 'Wireheads', *New Scientist* (5 January 2008), pp. 36–9.

19 Ehlers, A. and Clark, D.M., 'A cognitive model of post-traumatic stress disorder', *Behaviour Research and Therapy*, 38 (2000), pp. 319–45.

20 Burvil, P.W., 'Recent progress in the epidemiology of major depression', *Epidemiological Reviews*, Vol 17(1) (1995), pp. 21–31.

21 Lechin, F., Vanden Dijs, B. and Lechin, M.E., *Neurocircuitry and Neuroautonomic Disorders*, Karger (2002).

22 www.nimh.nih.gov

23 www.hc-sc.gc.ca

24 www.mcmanweb.com/article-200.htm

25 http://depression.about.com/cs/diagnosis/a/atypicaldepress.htm

26 Rose, S., 'Will science explain mental illness?', *Prospect*, issue 115 (October 2005).

27 www.sada.org.uk

28 Norman Rosenthal, *Winter Blues: Seasonal Affective Disorder: What it is and how to overcome it*, Guilford Press (1998).

29 Kraft, U., 'Lighten up', *Scientific American Mind* (November 2005).

30 Stein, A., 'Mother and Child', *Welcome News Supplement*, No 8 (2004); Beck, C.T., 'Predictors of postpartum depression: an update', *Nursing Research*, Vol 50 (2001), pp. 275–85.

31 Edhborg, M., 'The long-term impact of postnatal depressed mood on mothers + child interaction: a preliminary study', *Journal of Reproductive and Infant Psychology*, Vol 19 (2001), pp. 61–71; Field, T., et al, 'Pregnancy problems, postpartum depression, and early mother-infant interactions', *Developmental Psychology*, Vol 21 (1985), pp. 1152–6.

Chapter 3

1 Rita Carter, *Mapping the Mind*, Weidenfeld and Nicolson (1998).

2 Friedman, A., et al, 'Pyridostigmine brain penetration under stress enhances neuronal excitability and induces early immediate transcriptional response', *Nature Medicine*, Vol 2 (1996), pp. 1382–5; Hanin, I., 'The Gulf War, stress, and a leaky blood–brain barrier', *Nature Medicine*, Vol 2 (1996), pp. 1307–8; Ovadia, H., et al, 'Evaluation of the effect of stress on the blood–brain barrier: critical role of the brain perfusion time', *Brain Research*, Vol 905 (2001), pp. 21–5; Sinton, C.M., et al, 'Stressful manipulations that elevate corticosterone reduce blood–brain barrier permeability to pyridostigmine in the rat', *Toxicology and Applied Pharmacology*, Vol 165 (2000), pp. 99–105; Friedman, A. and Soreq, H., 'Stress may disturb the blood–brain barrier', *Nature Medicine*, Vol 2 (1996), pp. 1382–5.

3 de Vries, H.E., et al, 'The blood–brain barrier in neuroinflammatory diseases', *Pharmacology Review*, Vol 49 (1997), pp. 143–55.

4 Abou-Donia, M.B., et al, 'Increased neurotoxicity following concurrent exposure to pyidostigmine bromide, DEFT, and chlopyrifos', *Fundamental and Applied Toxicology*, Vol 34 (1996), pp. 201–22; Ashani, Y. and Catravas, G.N., 'Seizure-induced changes in the permeability of the blood–brain barrier following administration of anticholinesterase drugs to rats', *Biochemical Pharmacology*, Vol 30 (1981), pp. 2593–601.

5 Paul Maclean, *The triune brain in evolution*, Plenum Press (1990).

6 David Servan-Schreiber, *Healing without Freud or Prozac*, Rodale International (2005).

7 McDonald, A.J., 'Organization of amygdaloid projections to the prefrontal
   cortex and associated striatum in the rat', *Neuroscience*, Vol 44 (1991),
   pp. 1–14; Bechara, Q., et al, 'Different contribution of the human amygdala
   and ventromedial prefrontal cortex to decision-making', *Journal of
   Neuroscience*, Vol 19 (1999), pp. 5473–81.

8 Cahill, L., 'His brain, her brain', *Scientific American*, Vol 292(5) (2005), pp.
   40–7.

9 David Dobbs, 'Eric Kandel: From mind and brain and back', *Scientific
   American Mind*, Vol 33 (November 2007), pp. 33–7.

10 Herbert, J., et al, 'Do corticosteroids damage the brain?' *Journal of
   Neuroendocrinology*, Vol 18 (2006), pp. 393–411.

11 Maren, S. and Fanselow, M.S., 'The amygdala and fear conditioning: has the
   nut been cracked?' *Neuron*, Vol 16 (1996), pp. 237–40; McGaugh, J.L., 'The
   amygdala modulates the consolidation of memories of emotionally arousing
   experiences', *Annual Review of Neuroscience*, Vol 27 (2004), pp. 1–28; Liang,
   K.C., et al, 'The role of amygdala norepinephrine in memory formation:
   involvement of memory enhancing effect of peripheral epinephrine', *Chinese
   Journal of Physiology*, Vol 38 (1995), pp. 81–91.

12 Selye, H., 'A syndrome produced by diverse nocuous agents', *Nature* (1936);
   Selye, H., 'Diseases of adaptation', *Wisconsin Medical Journal*, Vol 49(6)
   (1950); Selye, H., 'Stress and the general adaptation syndrome', *British
   Medical Journal*, Vol 4667 (1950), pp. 1383–92; Selye, H., 'Stress and distress',
   Comprehensive Therapy, Vol 1 (1975), pp. 9–13.

13 Lechin, F., Vanden Dijs, B. and Lechin, M.E., *Neurocircuitry and
   Neuroautonomic Disorders*, Karger (2002).

14 Herbert, J., et al, 'Do corticosteroids damage the brain?' *Journal of
   Neuroendocrinology*, Vol 18 (2006), pp. 393–411.

15 Lechin, F., Vanden Dijs, B. and Lechin, M.E., *Neurocircuitry and
   Neuroautonomic Disorders*, Karger (2002).

Chapter 4

1 Goodyer, I.M., et al, 'Psychoendocrine antecedents of persistent first-episode
   major depression in adolescents: a community-based longitudinal enquiry',
   Psychological Medicine, Vol 33 (2003), pp. 601–10; Goodyer, I.M., et al,
   'Psychosocial and endocrine features of chronic first-episode major
   depression in 8–16 year olds', *Biological Psychiatry*, Vol 50 (2001), pp. 351–7.

2 Herbert, J., et al, 'Do corticosteroids damage the brain?' *Journal of
   Neuroendocrinology*, Vol 18 (2006), pp. 393–411.

3 Linkowski, P., et al, 'Twin study of the 24-h cortisol profile: evidence for
   genetic control of the human circadian clock', *American Journal of Physiology*,
   Vol 264 (1993), pp. E173–81; Wust, S., et al, 'Genetic factors, perceived
   chronic stress, and the free cortisol response to awakening',

Psychoneuroendocrinology, Vol 25 (2000), pp. 707–20.

4 David Dobbs, 'Eric Kandel: From mind and brain and back again', *Scientific American Mind*, Vol 33 (November 2007), pp. 33–7.

5 http://en.wikipedia.org/wiki/Epigenetics

6 Petronis, A., 'Epigenetics may account for 30–70 per cent of cases where only one twin has bipolar disorder', *American Journal of Medical Genetics* (November 2003).

7 Cahill, L., 'His brain, her brain', *Scientific American*, Vol 292(5) (2005), pp. 40–7; Hines, M., *Brain Gender*, Oxford University Press (2004); Seale, J.V., et al, 'Organizational role for testosterone and estrogen on adult hypothalamic-pituitary-adrenal axis activity in the male rat', *Endocrinology*, Vol 146 (2005), pp. 1973–82.

8 Windle, R.J., et al, 'The pulsatile characteristics of hypothalamo-pituitary-adrenal activity in female Lewis and Fischer 344 rats and its relationship to differential stress responses', *Endocrinology*, Vol 139 (1998), pp. 4044–52.

9 Seale, J.V., et al, 'Organizational role for testosterone and estrogen on adult hypothalamic-pituitary-adrenal axis activity in the male rat', *Endocrinology*, Vol 146 (2005), pp. 1973–1982.

10 Seckl, J.R., 'Prenatal glucocorticoids and long-term programming', *European Journal of Endocrinology*, Vol 1151 (Suppl 3) (2004), pp. U49–62.

11 Cahill, L., 'His brain, her brain', *Scientific American*, Vol 292(5) (2005), pp. 40–7.

12 Seckl, J.R., 'Prenatal glucocorticoids and long-term programming', *European Journal of Endocrinology*, Vol 1151 (Suppl 3) (2004), pp. U49–62; Dean, F., et al, 'Prenatal glucocorticoid modifies hypothalamo-pituitary-adrenal axis regulation in prepubertal guinea pigs', *Neuroendocrinology*, Vol 73 (2001), pp. 194–202; Nyirenda, M.J., et al, 'Programming hypoglycaemia in the rat through prenatal exposure to glucocorticoids – fetal effect or maternal influence?' *Journal of Endocrinology*, Vol 170 (2001), pp. 653–60.

13 Bhatnagar, S., et al, 'Prenatal stress differentially affects habituation of corticosterone responses to repeated stress in adult male and female rats', *Hormonal Behaviour*, Vol 47 (2005), pp. 430–8.

14 http://en.wikipedia.org/wiki/Social_cognition

15 Kathleen Kendall-Tackett, 'Post natal depression fought off by breastfeeding and good fats', www.medicalnewstoday.commedicalnews.php?newsid=69752

16 Liu, D., et al, 'Maternal care, hippocampal synaptogenesis and cognitive development in rats', *Nature Neuroscience*, Vol 3 (2000), pp. 799–806; Meaney, M.J., et al, 'Effect of neonatal handling on age-related impairments associated with the hippocampus', *Science*, Vol 239 (1988), pp. 766–8; Meaney, M.J., et al, 'Early environmental regulation of forebrain glucocorticoid receptor gene expression: implications for adrenocortical responses to stress', *Developmental Neuroscience*, Vol 18 (1996), pp. 49–72; Owen, D., et al,

'Maternal adversity, glucocorticoids and programming of neuroendocrine function and behaviour', *Neuroscience & Biobehavioral Reviews*, Vol 29 (2005), pp. 209–26.

17 Seckl, J.R., and Meaney, M.J., 'Glucocorticoid programming', *Annals of the New York Academy of Sciences*, Vol 1032 (2004), pp. 63–84; de Kloet, R.R., et al, 'Stress genes and the mechanism of programming the brain for later life', *Neuroscience & Biobehavioral Reviews*, Vol 29 (2005), pp. 271–81.

18 John Bowlby, *Attachment and Loss*, 3 vols (1969, 1973, 1980).

19 Kaufman, E.R., 'The intergenerational transmission of anxiety: a prospective study', Doctoral dissertation, The University of Texas at Austin (2003).

20 Allan Schore, *Affect Regulation and the Origin of the Self*, Lawrence Erlbaum (1999).

21 'Abnormal brain connectivity in children after early severe socioemotional deprivation: A Diffusion Tensor Imaging Study', *Pediatrics*, Vol 117(6) (June 2006), pp. 2093–100.

22 Hammen, C., et al, 'Intergenerational transmission of depression: test of interpersonal stress model in a community sample', *Journal of Consulting and Clinical Psychology*, Vol 72(3) (2004), pp. 511–22.

23 James, O., *They fuck you up: how to survive family life*, Bloomsbury (2003).

24 'Blame, insatiably demanding parents and our materialist society', Oliver James, Times 2, *The Times* (20 January 2006).

25 Quirarte, G.L., et al, 'Glucocorticoid enhancement of memory storage involves noradrenergic activation in the basolateral amygdala', *Proceedings of the National Academy of Sciences*, USA, Vol 94 (1997), pp. 14048–53; Mahew, F.S., et al, 'Differential effects of adrenergic and corticosteroid hormone systems on human short- and long-term declarative memory for emotionally arousing material', *Behavioural Neuroscience*, Vol 118 (2004), pp. 420–8.

26 www.rcpsych.ac.uk

27 Halligan, S.L., et al, 'Exposure to postnatal depression predicts elevated cortisol in adolescent offspring', *Biological Psychiatry*, Vol 55 (2004), pp. 811–15.

28 Martensz, N.D., et al, 'Relation between aggressive behaviour and circadian rhythms in cortisol and testosterone in social groups of talapoin monkeys', *Journal of Endocrinology*, Vol 115 (1987), pp. 107–20; Abbott, D.H., et al, 'Are subordinates always stressed? A comparative analysis of rank differences in cortisol levels among primates', *Hormones and Behavior*, Vol 43 (2003), pp. 67–82.

29 Lupien, S.J., et al, 'Child's stress hormone levels correlate with mother's socioeconomic status and depressive state', *Biological Psychiatry*, Vol 48 (2000), pp. 976–80; Lupien, S.J., et al, 'Can poverty get under your skin? Basal cortisol levels and cognitive function in children from low and high socioeconomic status', *Development and Psychopathology*, Vol 13 (2001), pp. 651–74.

30 Hellhammer, D.H., et al, 'Social hierarchy and adrenocortical stress reactivity in men', *Psychoneuroendocrinology*, Vol 22(8) (1997), pp. 643–50.

31 Marmot, M., 'Social determinants of health inequalities', *Lancet*, Vol 365 (2005), pp. 1099–104; Marmot, M., *Status Syndrome – how your social standing directly affects your health and life expectancy.* Bloomsbury Henry Holt (2004); Marmot, M.G., Davey Smith, G., Stansfeld, S., Patel, C., North, F., Head, J., White, I., Brunner, E. and Feeney, A., 'Health inequalities among British civil servants; the Whitehall II study', *Lancet*, Vol 337 (1991), pp. 1387–93; Marmot, M.G., Shipley, M.J. and Rose, G., 'Inequalities in death – specific explanations of a general pattern?' *Lancet* (1984), pp. 1003–6; Marmot, M.G., Adelstein, A.M., Robinson, N. and Rose, G., 'The changing social class distribution of heart disease', *BMJ* (1978) pp. 1109–12.

32 Pruessner, J.C., et al, 'Effects of self-esteem on age-related changes in cognition and the regulation of the hypothalamic-pituitary-adrenal axis', *Annals of the New York Academy of Sciences*, Vol 1032 (2004), pp. 186–94; Pruessner, J.C., et al, 'Self-esteem, locus of control, hippocampal volume, and cortisol regulation in young and old adulthood', *Neuroimage*, Vol 28 (2005), pp. 815–26.

33 'Blame, insatiably demanding parents and our materialist society', Oliver James, Times 2, *The Times* (20 January 2006).

34 Friedman, A., et al, 'Pyridostigmine brain penetration under stress enhances neuronal excitability and induces early immediate transcriptional response', *Nature Medicine*, Vol 2 (1996), pp. 1382–5; Hanin, I., 'The Gulf War, stress, and a leaky blood–brain barrier', *Nature Medicine*, Vol 2 (1996), pp. 1307–8.

35 Xun Song, et al, 'Interactive effects of paraoxon and pyridostigmine on blood–brain barrier integrity and cholinergic toxicity', *Toxicological Sciences*, 78 (2004), pp. 241–7.

36 Haorah, J., et al, 'Alcohol-induced oxidative stress in brain endothelial cells causes blood–brain barrier dysfunction', *Journal of Leucocyte Biology*, 78 (2005), pp. 1223–32.

37 Blaylock, R., *Excitotoxins, The taste that kills*, Health Press (1997).

38 Foster, H., 'How HIV-1 causes AIDS: implications for prevention and treatment', *Medical Hypotheses*, Vol 62(4), pp. 549–53.

39 Moore, T.M., et al, 'Cannabis use and risk of psychotic or affective mental health outcomes: a systematic review', *Lancet*, Vol 370 (2007), pp. 319–28.

40 Psychiatry.mc.duc.edu/Residents/substance.html; *Counselling & Psychotherapy Journal*, Vol 16(4) (May 2005), p. 27; www.aona.co.uk/addiction/cannabis /long-term-effects-brain

41 Johns, A., 'Psychiatric effects of cannabis', *British Journal of Psychiatry*, Vol 178 (2001), pp. 116–22.

42 *Sunday Times* (11 December 2005).

Chapter 5

1 Claire Ainsworth, 'Wireheads', *New Scientist* (5 January 2008), pp. 36–9.

2 Hall, R.C.W. (ed), *Psychiatric Presentations of Medical Illness*, SP Medical and Scientific Books (1980); Taylor, R.L., *Mind or Body: Distinguishing Psychological from Organic Disorder: Screening for Psychological Masquerade*, Springer Publishing (1990).

3 Diamond, R.J., 'Psychiatric presentations of medical illness' (2002), www.alternativementalhealth.com/articles/diamond.htm

4 'Drugs that cause psychiatric symptoms', *The Medical Letter* (23 July 1993).

5 Rethink (operating name of the UK National Schizophrenia Fellowship) Factsheet, *Getting a second opinion about diagnosis and/or treatment* (2003).

6 'Introduction to neurotransmitters', www.integrativemedonline.com/depressionandbrainchemistry.htm; 'Catecholamines – urine', www.umm.edu/ency/article/003613.htm; Leone, A.M., et al, 'The isolation, purification and characterisation of the principal urinary metabolites of melatonin', *Journal of Pineal Research*, Vol 4(3) (1987), pp. 253–66, www.ncbi.nlm.nih.gov; Tsuchiya, H., et al, 'High-performance liquid-chromatographic analysis for serotonin and tryptamine excreted in urine after oral loading with L-tryptophan', *Clin Chem*, Vol 35(1) (1989), pp. 43–7; Lechin, F., Vanden Dijs, B. and Lechin, M.E., *Neurocircuitry & Neuroautonomic Disorders*, Karger (2002) and references therein.

7 Melichar, J. and Donaldson, L., 'Taste buds respond differently to depression therapies that target serotonin and noradrenaline', *Journal of Neuroscience* (2006).

8 Netherton, C., et al, 'Salivary cortisol and dehydroepiandrosterone in relation to puberty and gender', *Psychoneuroendocrinology*, Vol 29 (2004), pp. 125–40; Putignano, P., et al, Salivary cortisol measurement in normal-weight, obese and anorexic women: comparison with plasma cortisol, *European Journal of Endocrinology*, Vol 145(2) (2001), pp. 165–71.

9 Fuchs, E., et al, 'Salivary cortisol: a non-invasive measure of hypothalamo-pituitary-adrenocortical activity in the squirrel monkey, *Saimiri sciureus*', *Laboratory Animals*, Vol 31(4) (1997), pp. 306–11.

10 Shively, C.A., 'Brain scans show depressed monkeys have same central-nervous system characteristics as people', *Archives of General Psychiatry* (April 2006).

11 Crook, I., 'Scan predicts path of depression', *BBC News Health* (June 2002).

12 Sherman, D., 'Super Bowl ads fumble, brain scans show', *Guardian Unlimited* (2007).

13 www.time.com/time/Europe/magazine/2002/0826/anxiety/story3.html

14 Holman, B.L. and Devous, M.D., 'Functional brain SPECT: the emergence of a powerful clinical method', *Journal of Nuclear Medicine*, Vol 33 (1992), pp. 1888–904.

15 Juni, J.E., et al, 'Procedure guideline for brain perfusion SPECT using technetium-99m radiopharmaceuticals', *Journal of Nuclear Medicine*, Vol 39 (1998), pp. 923–6; Raine, A., et al, 'Reduced prefrontal and increased subcortical brain functioning assessed using positron emission tomography in predatory and affective murderers', *Behavioral Sciences and the Law*, Vol 16 (1998), pp. 319–32; Volkow, N.D. and Tancredi, L., 'Neural substrates of violent behavior: A preliminary study with positron emission tomography', *British Journal of Psychiatry*, Vol 151 (1987), pp. 668–73; Tiihonen, J., et al, 'Single-photon emission tomography imaging of monoamine transporters in impulsive violent behaviour', *European Journal of Nuclear Medicine*, Vol 24 (1997), pp. 1253–60; Nicolas, J.M., et al, 'Regional cerebral blood flow-SPECT in chronic alcoholism: relation to neuropsychological testing', *Journal of Nuclear Medicine*, Vol 34 (1993), pp. 1452–9; Amen, D.G. and Waugh, M., 'High resolution brain SPECT imaging of marijuana smokers with AD/HD', *Journal of Psychoactive Drugs*, Vol 30 (1998), pp. 209–14.

16 Amen, D.G. and Routh, L.C., *Healing anxiety and depression*, Berkley Trade (2004).

17 Datz, F.L., et al, *Nuclear Medicine: A Teaching File*, Mosby (1992), p. 220.

18 'Can brain scans see depression?', *New York Times* (18 October 2005).

19 Lechin, F., Vanden Dijs, B. and Lechin, M.E., *Neurocircuitry & Neuroautonomic Disorders*, Karger (2002) and references therein.

20 Jane Plant and Gill Tidey, *The Plant Programme*, Virgin Books (2002).

Chapter 6

1 *Chemical & Engineering News*, Vol 81 (2003), pp. 22, 33–7.

2 http://en.wikipedia.org/wiki/Tricyclic_antidepressant

3 Cade, J.F.J., 'Lithium salts in the treatment of psychotic excitement', *Med J Aust* (1949), pp. 349–52.

4 Dawson, E.B., 'The relationship of tap water and physiological levels of lithium to mental hospital admission and homicide in Texas', in *Lithium in Biology and Medicine*, Schrauzer, G.N. and Klippel, K.F. (eds), VCH Verlag (1991), pp. 171–87.

5 Lechin, F., Vanden Dijs, B. and Lechin, M.E., *Neurocircuitry & Neuroautonomic Disorders*, Karger (2002) and references therein.

6 www.benzo.org.uk/behan.htm; www.benzos.net; www.aafp.org/afp/20000401/2121.html; www.tranx.org.au/benzodiaz.html

7 www.drug-concern.co.uk/dconcern/classc.php

8 Timmons, C.R. and Hamilton, L.W., www.rci.rutgers.edu/~lwh/drugs/

9 *Counselling and Psychotherapy Journal*, Vol 16(4) (May 2005).

10 'Introduction to neurotransmitters',
www.integrativemedonline.com/depressionandbrainchemistry.htm

11 Sandyk, R., 'L-Tryptophan in neuro psychiatric disorders, a review', *Int J Neuroscience*, Vol 67 (1992), pp. 24–144; Young, S.N. and Teff, K.L., 'Tryptophan availability, 5HTP synthesis and 5HT function', *Prog Neuro Psychopharmacol and Bio Psychiat*, Vol 13 (1989), pp. 173–9.

12 Kelly, G.S., '*Rodiola rosea*: a possible plant adaptogen', *Alternative Medical Reviews*, Vol 6(3) (2001), pp. 293–302.

13 Bartram, T., *Bartram's encyclopaedia of Herbal Medicine*, Constable (1995).

14 Bartram, T., *Bartram's encyclopaedia of Herbal Medicine*, Constable (1995); Ernst, E., *The Desktop Guide to Complementary and Alternative Medicine, an evidence based approach*, Mosby (2001).

15 Ernst, E., *The Desktop Guide to Complementary and Alternative Medicine, an evidence based approach*, Mosby (2001).

16 Berman, R.M., et al, 'Antidepressant effects of ketamine in depressed patients', *Biological Psychiatry*, Vol 47(4) (2000), pp. 351–4; Akira Kudoh, et al, 'Small-dose ketamine improves the post-operative state of depressed patients', *Anesthesia and Analgesia*, Vol 95 (2002) , pp. 114–18; Sanacora, G., et al, 'Subtype-specific alterations of gamma-aminobutyric acid and glutamate in patients with major depression', *Archives in General Psychiatry*, Vol 61(7) (2004), pp. 705–13; Zarate, C.A., et al, 'A randomised trial of an *N*-methyl-D-aspartate antagonist in treastment-resistant major depression', *Archives in General Psychiatry* Vol 63(8) (2006), pp. 856–64.

Chapter 7

1 *Talking treatments and psychological therapies*, Rethink (National Schizophrenia Fellowship) (2003).

2 *The Depression Report: A New Deal for Depression and Anxiety Disorders*. A report by The Centre for Economic Performance's Mental Health Policy Group, The London School of Economics & Political Science.

3 David Dobbs, 'Eric Kandel: From mind and brain and back again', *Scientific American Mind*, Vol 33 (November 2007), pp. 33–7.

4 *The Depression Report: A New Deal for Depression and Anxiety Disorders*. A report by The Centre for Economic Performance's Mental Health Policy Group, The London School of Economics & Political Science.

5 Colin Feltham, *Introduction to counselling and psychotherapy*, Sage Publications (2006), p. 5.

6 The Westminster Pastoral Foundation, www.wpf.org.uk

7 Beck, A.,'Cognitive Therapy: a 30 year retrospective', *American Psychology*, Vol 46 (1991), pp. 368–75.

8 Peter McGuffin, 'Will science explain mental illness? Yes', *Prospect* (October 2005).

9 Dobbs D., 'Eric Kandel: From mind and brain and back again', *Scientific American Mind*, Vol 33 (November 2007), pp. 33–7.

10 Dobbs, D., 'Turning off Depression', *Scientific American Mind* (2006).

11 Arkowitz, H. and Lilienfeld, S., 'A pill to fix your ills?' *Scientific American Mind* (February/March 2007).

12 Carl Rogers, *On Becoming a Person*, Constable & Robinson (1961).

13 David Servan-Schreiber, *Healing Without Freud or Prozac*, Rodale International (2005).

14 Ernst, E., *The Desktop Guide to Complementary and Alternative Medicine, an evidence based approach*, Mosby (2001).

15 Beales, D., 'Beyond mind–body dualism: implications for patient care', *Journal of Holistic Health Care*, Vol 1 (2004).

16 Biello, D., 'Searching for God in the Brain', *Scientific American Mind*, Vol 33 (November 2007), pp. 39–45.

17 Beales, D., 'Beyond mind–body dualism: implications for patient care', *Journal of Holistic Health Care*, Vol 1 (2004).

18 David Servan-Schreiber, *Healing Without Freud or Prozac*, Rodale International (2005).

19 Lilienfeld, S.O. and Arkowitz, H., 'Taking a closer look', *Scientific American Mind* (December 2006 /January 2007).

20 Shapiro, F., *Eye movement desensitization and reprocessing: Basic principles, protocols, and procedures*, Guilford Press (1995).

21 Devilly, G.J., 'Eye movement desensitization and reprocessing: a chronology of its development and scientific standing', *Scientific Review of Mental Health Practice*, Vol 1, (2002) pp. 113–38.

22 Westerhoff, N., 'Fantasy Therapy', *Scientific American Mind*, (October/November 2007), pp. 71–5.

23 Ernst, E., *The Desktop Guide to Complementary and Alternative Medicine, an evidence based approach*, Mosby (2001).

24 Kent, H., *The Complete Illustrated Guide to Yoga*, Element (1999); Ernst, E., *The Desktop Guide to Complementary and Alternative Medicine, an evidence based approach*, Mosby (2001).

Chapter 8

1 Andre, L., 'Testimony at the public hearing of the New York State (U.S.) Assembly Standing Committee on Mental Health on electroconvulsive therapy', (2001); Cameron, D.G., 'ECT: sham statistics, the myth of convulsive therapy, and the case for consumer misinformation', *J Mind Behav*, Vol 15 (1994), pp. 177–98.

2 en.wikipedia.org/wiki/Electroconvulsive.therapy

3 McGregor-Robertson, J., *The Household Physician*, Blackie & Son (1890).

4 serendip.brynmawr.edu/bb/neuro00/web2/Hollander.html

5 Diehl, D.J., et al, 'Post-ECT increases in T2 relaxation times and their relationship to cognitive side effects: a pilot study', *Psychiatry Res*, Vol 54 (1994).

6 en.wikipedia.org/wiki/Electroconvulsive.therapy

7 http://psychirights.org

8 Corsellis, J. and Meyer, A., 'Histological changes in the brain after uncomplicated electro-convulsive treatment', *J Mental Sci*, Vol 100 (1954), pp. 375–83; Ebaugh, F.G., et al, 'Fatalities following electric convulsive therapy. A report of two cases with autopsy findings', *Trans Am Neurol Assoc*, Vol 36 (1942); Ferraro, A., et al, 'Morphologic changes in the brains of monkeys following convulsions electrically induced', *J Neuropathol Exp Neurol*, Vol 5 (1946), p. 285; Janis, I.L., 'Psychologic effects of electric convulsive treatments. I: Post-treatment amnesias', *J Nervous Mental Dis*, Vol 111 (1950), pp. 359–81.

9 Behrman, A., *Electroboy: A Memoir of Mania*, Random House (2005).

10 Christine Toomey and Steven Young, 'Mental Cruelty', *Sunday Times Magazine* (19 February 2006).

11 Basant Puri, *Attention-Deficit Hyperactivity Disorder: a natural way to treat ADHD*, Hammersmith Press (2005); David Servan-Schreiber, *Healing Without Freud or Prozac*, Rodale International (2005).

12 Schulze-Rauschenbach, S.C., et al, 'Distinctive neurocognitive effects of repetitive transcranial magnetic stimulation and electroconvulsive therapy in major depression', *British Journal of Psychiatry*, Vol 186 (2005), pp. 410–16.

13 Claire Ainsworth, 'Wireheads', *New Scientist* (5 January 2008), pp. 36–9.

14 Christine Toomey and Steven Young, 'Mental Cruelty', *Sunday Times Magazine* (19 February 2006).

15 Claire Ainsworth, 'Wireheads', *New Scientist* (5 January 2008), pp. 36–9.

16 Dobbs, D., 'Turning off Depression', *Scientific American Mind* (2006).

17 Claire Ainsworth, 'Wireheads', *New Scientist* (5 January 2008), pp. 36–9

18 Kraft, U., 'Lighten Up', *Scientific American Mind*, November 2005.

Chapter 9

1 Matthew Johnstone, *I had a black dog*, Constable and Robinson (2007).

2 www.who.int/mental_health/prevention/suicide/suiciderates/en

3 De Vries, Jan, lecture Rude Health Show, Dublin, September 2007.

4 Jones, D., 'Going global', *New Scientist* (27 October 2007), pp. 36–41.

5 Basant Puri, *Attention-Deficit Hyperactivity Disorder: a natural way to treat ADHD*, Hammersmith Press (2005); David Servan-Schreiber, *Healing without Freud or Prozac*, Rodale International (2005).

6 Biello, D., 'Searching for God in the Brain', *Scientific American Mind*, Vol 33 (November 2007), pp. 39–45.

7 Jones, D., 'Going global', *New Scientist* (27 October 2007), pp. 36–41.

8 Reilly, M., 'God's place in a rational world', *New Scientist* (10 November 2007).

9 Henry Haslam, *The Moral Mind*, Imprint Academic (2005).

10 Dubler and Gurel, 'Depression: relationships to clothing and appearance self-concept', *Family and Consumer Sciences Research Journal*, Vol 13 (1984), pp. 21–6; Davison, T. and McCabe, N., 'Relationships between men's and women's body image and their psychological, social and sexual functioning', *Sex roles*, Vol 52(7–8) (2005), pp. 463–75.

11 *The Real Truth About Beauty: A Global Report*, commissioned by Dove (2004).

12 David Servan-Schreiber, *Healing Without Freud or Prozac*, Rodale International (2005).

13 Lewis Wolpert, *Malignant Sadness, the Anatomy of Depression*, 3rd edition, Faber & Faber (2006).

14 Burton, R., *The Anatomy of Melancholy* (1651), ed Faulkner et al, Clarendon Press (1989–94).

15 *The Depression Report: A New Deal for Depression and Anxiety Disorders*. A report by The Centre for Economic Performance's Mental Health Policy Group, The London School of Economics & Political Science.

16 For example, www.richmond.cvs.org.uk

17 Mathews, V., 'Video Game Violence Goes Straight to Kids' Heads', Indiana University School of Medicine, ScoutNews LLC (2006).

18 Darius Leszczynski, quoted by James Meek in the *Guardian* (20 June 2002).

19 Ernst, E., *The Desktop Guide to Complementary and Alternative Medicine, an evidence based approach*, Mosby (2001).

20 Wenner M., 'Exercising generates new brain cells', *Scientific American Mind*, (June/July 2007), p. 10; Branan, N. '… And stress kills them off', *Scientific American Mind* (June/July 2007), p. 10.

21 www.mentalhealth.org.nz

22 Ernst, E., *The Desktop Guide to Complementary and Alternative Medicine, an evidence based approach*, Mosby (2001).

23 Frumkin, H., Frank, L. and Jackson, R., *Urban Sprawl and Public Health 2004*, Island Press (2004).

24 Royal Commission on Environmental Pollution, *The Urban Environment* (2007).

25 Kunstler, J., *Big and Blue in the USA*, Orion Online (2003).

26 Department of Health and Human Services (US), *Healthy People 2010*, Volume 1. DHHS (November 2000).

27 Bill Bryson, *Notes from a Small Island*, Doubleday (1995).

28 Frumkin, H., Frank, L. and Jackson, R., *Urban Sprawl and Public Health 2004*, Island Press (2004).

29 Ulrich, R.S., 'View through a window may influence recovery from surgery', *Science*, Vol 224 (1984), pp. 420–1.

30 David Rose, 'Walking and work therapy could help millions throw away the pills', *The Times* (14 May 2007).

31 Maller, C., Townsend, M., Brown, P. and St Leger, L., *Healthy Parks, Healthy People: the health benefits of contact with nature in a park context: a review of current literature*, Deakin University and Parks, Victoria, Australia (2002); Stone, D. and Hanna, J., 'Health and Nature: the sustainable option for healthy cities', Paper presented at the Healthy Cities Conference, Belfast (2003).

32 Ineichen, B., *Homes and Health: how housing and health interact*, Spon (1993).

33 Barnes, S., 'A grassroots remedy', *The Times* (11 June 2007).

34 Grandjean, P. and Landrigan, P.J., 'Developmental neurotoxicity of industrial chemicals', www.thelancet.com, published online 8 November, 2006; Grandjean, P. and Perez, M., 'Potentials for exposure to industrial chemicals suspected of causing developmental neurotoxicity', appendix to Grandjean, P. and Landrigan, P.J., 'Developmental neurotoxicity of industrial chemicals', www.thelancet.com, published online 8 November 2006.

35 www.panda.org/about_wwf/where_we_work/europe/what_we_do/epo /index.cfm?uNewsID=9941

36 Goyer, A. and Clarkson, T.W., 'Toxic effects of metals', in *Cassarett and Doull's Toxicology. The Basic Science of Poisons*. Klaassen, C.D. (ed), McGraw-Hill (2001), pp. 811–68.

37 Hrdina, P.D., et al, 'Effects of chronic exposure to cadmium, lead and mercury of brain biogenic amines in the rat', *Research Communications in Chemical Pathology and Pharmacology*, Vol 15(3) (1976), pp. 483–93.

38 www.vaccineinfo.net/immunization/injury/autism/DanishMMRAutismStudy .shtml; www.cdc.gov/od/science/iso/concerns/thimerosal.htm

39 www.fsan.fda.gov/-frf/sea-mehg.html; www.food.gov.uk/multimedia/faq/mercuryfish/

40 Editorial in *Chemical and Engineering News*, Vol 81(22), pp. 33–7.

41 Gottesfeld, Z., 'Effect of lithium and other alkali metals on brain chemistry and behaviour. I Glutamic acid and GABA in brain regions', *Psychopharmacologia*, Vol 45(2) (1976), pp. 239–42.

42 Stenersen, J., *Chemical Pesticides*, CRC Press (2004).

43 Adams, M.D., et al, 'The genome sequence of *Drosophila melanogaster*', *Science*, Vol 287 (2000), pp. 2185–95; Royal Commission on Environmental Pollution, Twenty-fifth Report – 'Turning the Tide: Addressing the Impact of Fisheries on the Marine Environment' (December 2004).

44 Davis, D.R., et al., 'Chronic exposure to organophosphates: background and clinical picture', *Advances in Psychiatric Treatment*, Vol 6 (2000), pp. 187–92.

45 Stenersen, J., *Chemical Pesticides*, CRC Press (2004).

46 'Crop Spraying and the Health of Residents and Bystanders', Royal Commission on Environmental Pollution, Special Report (2005).

Chapter 10

1 Jeffery, D.R., 'Nutrition and diseases of the nervous system', in *Modern Nutrition in Health and Disease*, 9th edition, Shils, M.E., et al (eds), Williams and Wilkins (1999); Westermarck, T. and Antila, E., 'Diet in relation to the nervous system', in *Human Nutrition and Dietetics*, 10th edition, Garrow, J.S., et al (eds), Churchill Livingstone (2000).

2 Alexandra Massey, *SuperFoods*, Virgin Books (2006).

3 FDA – USA, 'Mercury Levels in Commercial Fish and Shellfish', www.fsan.fda.gov/-frf/sea-mehg.html; FSA – UK: 2002, Position on fish consumption, www.orpha.onca/ppres/2004-04_pp.pdf

4 Courtney Van de Weyer, *Changing Diets, Changing Minds: how food affects mental well-being and behaviour*, Sustain and the Mental Health Foundation (2005).

5 Patrick Holford, *Optimum Nutrition for the Mind*, Piatkus (2004).

6 Campbell, T. and Campbell, T.M., *The China Study*, Benbella Books (2006); Jane Plant, *Your Life in Your Hands: Understand, Prevent and Overcome Breast Cancer and Ovarian Cancer*, 4th edition, Virgin Books (2007); John Robbins, *Diet for a New America*, H.J. Kramer (1987).

7 Stinson, S., 'Early Childhood Health in Foragers', in *The Human Diet: Its Origin and Evolution*, ed. Ungar, P. S. and Teaford, M.F., Bergin & Garvey (2002); Tansey, G. and Worsley, T., *The Food System: A Guide*, Earthscan (1995).

8 Tudge, C., *So Shall We Reap: How Everyone Who is Liable to be Born in the Next Ten Thousand Years Could Eat Very Well Indeed: and Why, in Practice, Our Immediate Descendants Are Likely to Be in Serious Trouble*, Allen Lane (2003).

9 Eaton, S.B., et al, 'Evolution, Diet and Health', in *The Human Diet: Its Origins*

and Evolution, ed Ungar, P.S. and Teaford, M.F., Bergin & Garvey (2002).

10 Hibbeln, J., Speech to the Associate Parliamentary Food and Health Forum, London (2003).

11 Larsen, C.S., 'Dietary Reconstruction and Nutritional Assessment of Past Peoples: The Bioanthropological Record', in *The Cambridge World History of Food*, ed Kiple, K. F. and Ornelas, K.C., Cambridge University Press (2000); Eaton, S.B., et al, Evolution, Diet and Health', in *The Human Diet: Its Origins and Evolution*, ed Ungar, P.S. and Teaford, M.F., Bergin & Garvey (2002); Tansey, G. and Worsley, T., *The Food System: A Guide*, Earthscan (1995).

12 Cohen, M.N., 'History, Diet, and Hunter-Gatherers', in *The Cambridge World History of Food*, ed Kiple, K. F. and Ornelas, K. C., Cambridge University Press (2000), pp. 63–71.

13 Tansey, G. and Worsley, T., *The Food System: A Guide*, Earthscan (1995).

14 Courtney Van de Weyer, *Changing Diets, Changing Minds: how food affects mental well-being and behaviour*, Sustain and the Mental Health Foundation (2005).

15 Marion Nestle, *Food Politics: How the Food Industry Influences Nutrition and Health*, Berkeley, University of California Press (2002).

16 Defra, *Family Food – Report on the Expenditure and Food Survey*, National Statistics (2005).

17 *Organic Food: Facts and Figures*, Soil Association (December 2004); Pesticides in Your Food; Andy Jones, *Eating Oil: food supply in a changing climate*, Sustain (2001).

18 Small, M.F., 'The Happy Fat', *New Scientist* (24 August 2002).

19 Eaton, S.B., et al,. 'Evolution, Diet and Health', in *The Human Diet: Its Origins and Evolution*, ed Ungar, P.S. and Teaford, M.F., Bergin & Garvey (2002).

20 Philip Conford, *The Origins of the Organic Movement*, Floris Books (2001).

21 Courtney Van de Weyer, *Changing Diets, Changing Minds: how food affects mental well-being and behaviour*, Sustain and the Mental Health Foundation (2005).

22 Butler, J., *White Lies: The Health Consequences of Consuming Cows Milk*, Vegetarian and Vegan Foundation (2006).

23 Mayer, A.B., 'Historical Changes in the Mineral Content of Fruit and Vegetables', *British Food Journal*, Vol 99(6) (1997); Thomas, D.E., 'Study on the Mineral Depletion of the Foods Available to us as a Nation over the Period 1940 to 1991', *Nutrition and Health*, Vol 17(2) (2003); Farewell, T.S., *Summary of Change of Zinc and Magnesium in Soils across England and Wales*, National Soil Resources Institute (NSRI), Cranfield University at Silsoe (2005).

24 *Pesticides in Your Food*, Pan-UK (2004).

25 Annual Report of the Pesticide Residues Committee (2002); RCEP pesticides short report.

26 Annual Report of the Pesticide Residues Committee (2002); RCEP pesticides short report; Annual Report of the Pesticide Residues Committee (2002).

27 Annual Report of the Pesticide Residues Committee (2002).

28 Royal Commission on Environmental Pollution, Twenty-fifth Report – 'Turning the Tide: Addressing the Impact of Fisheries on the Marine Environment' (Presented to Parliament by Command of Her Majesty) (December 2004).

29 Lucy Yates, *Greener?* National Consumer Council (2007).

30 Lu, C., et al, 'Organic diets significantly lower children's dietary exposure to organophosphorus pesticides', *Environmental Health Perspectives*, Vol 114(2) (2006), pp. 260–3.

31 Tansey, G. and Worsley, T., *The Food System: A Guide*, Earthscan (1995).

32 Boyle, C., *European Food Facts and Figures*, Leatherhead Food RA: Market Intelligence Section (2000).

33 Courtney Van de Weyer, *Changing Diets, Changing Minds: how food affects mental well-being and behaviour*, Sustain and the Mental Health Foundation (2005).

34 John Humphrys, *The Great Food Gamble*, Coronet Books (2002).

35 Blaylock, R., *Excitotoxins, The taste that kills*, Health Press (1997).

36 Mattes, J.A. and Gittelman, R., 'Effects of artificial food colourings in children with hyperactive symptoms', *Arch Gen Psychiatry*, Vol 38(6) (1981), pp. 714–18; David, T.J., 'Reactions to dietary tartrazine', *Archives of disease in childhood*, Vol 62 (1987), pp. 119–22.

37 Nutrition and mental health, www.minddisorders.com/kau-Nu/Nutition-and-mental-health.html; D Amour, M.L. and Butterworth, R.F., 'Pathogenesis of alcoholic peripheral neuropathy: direct effect of ethanol or nutritional deficit?' *Metab Brain Dis* (1994), pp. 133–42; Anderson, I.M., et al, 'Dieting reduces plasma tryptophan and alters brain 5-HT function in women', *Psychological Medicine*, Vol 20 (1990), pp. 785–91; Wurtman, R.J. and Wurtman, J.J., 'Brain serotonin, carbohydrate-craving, obesity and depression', *Obesity Research*, Vol 3 (1995), pp. 477S–80S; Goodwin, G.M., 'Plasma concentrations of tryptophan and dieting', *British Medical Journal*, Vol 300 (1990), pp. 1499–1500; Schweigger, U., et al, 'Macronutrient intake, plasma large neutral amino acids and mood during weight-reducing diets', *Journal of Neural Transmission*, Vol 67 (1986), pp. 77–86.

38 Campbell, T.C. and Campbell, T.M., *The China Study*, Benbella Books (2006).

39 Keith, R.E., et al, 'Alterations in dietary carbohydrate, protein and fat intake and mood state in trained female cyclists', *Medicine and Science in Sports and Exercise*, Vol 23(2) (1991), pp. 212–16.

40 Jane Plant and Gill Tidey, *Eating For Better Health*, Virgin Books (2001).

41 Fox, D., 'Hard Cheese', *New Scientist* (15 December 2001), pp. 42–5.

42 Jane Plant and Gill Tidey, *Osteoporosis*, Virgin Books (2003) and references therein.

43 Small, M.F., 'The Happy Fat', *New Scientist* (24 August 2002).

44 Butler, J., *White Lies: The Health Consequences of Consuming Cows Milk*, Vegetarian and Vegan Foundation (2006).

45 Tim Lang and Michael Heasman, *Food Wars: The Battle for Mouths, Minds and Markets*, Earthscan Publications (2004).

46 Crawford, M. and Marsh, D., *The Driving Force: Food in Evolution and The Future*, Mandarin (1989).

47 Michael Crawford, *What We Eat Today*, Spearman (1972).

48 Clover, C., *The End of the Line: How Overfishing is Changing the World and What We Eat*, Ebury Press (2004).

49 Puri, B.K., *Attention Deficit Hyperactivity Disorder*, Hammersmith Press (2005).

50 Small, M.F., 'The Happy Fat', *New Scientist* (24 August 2002).

51 Puri, B.K., *Attention Deficit Hyperactivity Disorder*, Hammersmith Press (2005).

52 Small, M.F., 'The Happy Fat', *New Scientist* (24 August 2002).

53 Puri, B.K., *Attention Deficit Hyperactivity Disorder*, Hammersmith Press (2005).

54 Royal Commission on Environmental Pollution, Twenty-fifth Report – 'Turning the Tide: Addressing the Impact of Fisheries on the Marine Environment' (Presented to Parliament by Command of Her Majesty) (December 2004).

55 Menkes, D.B., et al, 'Acute tryptophan depletion aggravates premenstrual syndrome', *J Affect Disord*, Vol 3291 (1994), pp. 37–44.

56 Willett, W.C. and Stamfer, M.J., 'Rebuilding the food pyramid', *Scientific American Reports*, Vol 16(4) (2006), pp. 12–21.

57 Yudkin, John S., *Pure, White and Deadly: Problem of sugar*, Davis-Poynter (1972).

58 Puri, B.K., *Attention Deficit Hyperactivity Disorder*, Hammersmith Press (2005).

59 Jane Plant and Gill Tidey, *The Plant Programme*, Virgin Books (2004); Campbell, T. and Campbell, T.M., *The China Study*, Benbella Books (2006); Eaton, S.B., et al, 'Evolution, Diet and Health', in *The Human Diet: Its Origins and Evolution*, ed Ungar, P.S. and Teaford, M.F., Bergin & Garvey (2002).

60 Jane Plant and Gill Tidey, *Eating for Better Health*, Virgin Books (2005); Campbell, T. and Campbell, T.M., *The China Study*, Benbella Books (2006); Eaton, S.B., et al, 'Evolution, Diet and Health', in *The Human Diet: Its Origins and Evolution*, ed Ungar, P.S. and Teaford, M.F., Bergin & Garvey (2002).

61 Campbell, T. and Campbell, T.M., *The China Study*, Benbella Books (2006).

62 Jane Plant and Gill Tidey, *The Plant Programme*, Virgin Books (2004); Jane Plant and Gill Tidey, *Eating for Better Health*, Virgin Books (2005); Robbins, J.,

The Food Revolution: How Your Diet Can Save Your Life and Our World, Red Wheel (2001); Robbins, J., *Diet for a New America*, H.J. Kramer (1987); Campbell, T. and Campbell, T.M., *The China Study*, Benbella Books (2006).

63 Campbell, T. and Campbell, T.M., *The China Study*, Benbella Books (2006).

64 Caine, D., Halliday, G.M., Kril, J.J. and Harper, C.G., 'Operational criteria for the classification of chronic alcoholics: identification of Wernicke's encephalopathy', *J. Neurol Neurosurg Psychiatry*, Vol 62 (1997), pp. 51–60.

65 Molina, J.A., Bermejo, F., del Ser, T., et al, 'Alcohol cognitive deterioration and nutritional deficiencies', *Acta Neurol Scand*, Vol 89 (1994), pp. 384–90.

66 Leklem, J.E., 'Vitamin B6', in *Modern Nutrition in Health and Disease*, 9th edition, Shils, M.E., et al (eds), Williams and Wilkins (1999), pp. 413–21.

67 Jo Steele, 'Depressed? A bit of dirt could help?' *Metro* (2 April 2007).

68 Schrauzer, G.N., 'Lithium: occurrence, dietary intakes, nutritional essentiality', *Journal of the American College of Nutrition*, Vol 21(1) (2002), pp. 14–21; Schrauzer, G.N., et al, 'Lithium in scalp hair of adults, students and violent criminals', *Biol Trace El Res*, Vol 34 (1992), pp. 161–76; Anke, M., et al, 'The biological importance of lithium', in *Lithium in Biology and Medicine*, Schrauzer, G.N. and Klippel, K.F. (eds), VCH Verlag (1991), pp. 149–67; Anke, M., et al, 'Evidence for the essentiality of lithium in goats', in *Proceedings 4. Spurenelement Symposium 1983*, Anke, M., et al (eds), VEB Kongressdruck (1983), pp. 58–65; Ono, T. and Wada, O., 'Effect of lithium deficient diet on avoidance behavior of animals and a discussion of the essentiality of lithium', *Biomed Res Trace El*, Vol 2 (1991), pp. 264–5; Dawson, E.B., et al, 'Relationship of lithium metabolism to mental hospital admission and homicide', *Dis Nerv Syst*, Vol 33 (1972), pp. 546–56; Schrauzer, G.N. and de Vroey, E., 'Effects of nutritional lithium supplementation on mood', *Biol Trace El*, Vol 40 (1994), pp. 89–101.

69 Puri, B.K., *Attention Deficit Hyperactivity Disorder*, Hammersmith Press (2005); Small, M.F., 'The Happy Fat', *New Scientist* (24 August 2002).

70 www.who.int/mental_health/prevention/suicide/suiciderates/en

71 *Annals of Internal Medicine* (1 July 2003); www.nlm.nih.gov/medlineplus/news/fullstory_13210.html; Bender, D.A., 'Daily doses of multivitamin tablets', *BMJ*, Vol 325 (2002), pp. 173–4.

72 Foster, H.D., 'Aids and "selenium – CDR T cell tailspin": the geography of a pandemic', *Townsend letter for doctors and patients*, 209 (2000), pp. 94–9.

73 Meyers, S., 'Use of neurotransmitter precursors for treatment of depression', *Altern Med Rev*, Vol 5(1) (2000), pp. 64–71.

74 Lamb, S., 'Precursor loading for monoamines in neurological disease', *Journal of Neurosurgical Nursing*, Vol 4 (15 August 1983), pp. 228–33; Young, V.R. and Ajami, A.M., 'Glutamate: an amino acid of particular distinction', *Journal of Nutrition*, Vol 130 (2000), pp. 892S–900S; 'Behavioural effects of dietary neurotransmitter precursors: basic and clinical aspects', *Neuroscience and Behavioral Reviews*, Vol 20(2) (1996), pp. 313–23; Chiaroni, P., et al, 'A

multivariate analysis of red blood cell membrane transports and plasma levels of L-tyrosine and L-tryptophan in depressed patients before treatment and after clinical improvement', *Neuropsychobiology*, Vol 23(1) (1990), pp. 1–7; Fernstrom, J.D., 'Can nutrient supplements modify brain function?' *American Journal of Clinical Nutrition*, Vol 71(6 Suppl) (2000), pp. 1669S–75S.

75 Groff, J.L. and Gropper, S.S., et al, *Advanced nutrition and human metabolism*, 3rd edition, West Publishing Company (1999).

76 Fernstrom, M.H. and Fernstrom, J.D., 'Brain tryptophan concentrations and serotonin synthesis remain responsive to food consumption after the ingestion of sequential meals', *American Journal of Clinical Nutrition*, Vol 61(2) (1995), pp. 312–19.

77 Giacometti, T., 'Free and bound glutamate in natural products', *Advances in Biochemistry and Physiology* (1979).

78 Salminen, R. (chief ed), *Geochemical Atlas of Europe*, FOREGS (2005).

79 Kolpin, D.A., et al, 'Pharmaceuticals, hormones and other organic wastewater contaminants in US streams, 1999–2000: a national reconnaissance', *Environmental Science & Technology*, Vol 36 (2002), pp. 1202–11.

Chapter 11

1 UK Psychiatric Morbidity Survey, 2000.

2 *The Depression Report: A New Deal for Depression and Anxiety Disorders*, A report by The Centre for Economic Performance's Mental Health Policy Group, The London School of Economics & Political Science, *Observer* (18 June 2006).

3 Lewis Wolpert, *Malignant Sadness, the Anatomy of Depression*, 3rd edition, Faber & Faber (2006).

4 *The Depression Report: A New Deal for Depression and Anxiety Disorders*, A report by The Centre for Economic Performance's Mental Health Policy Group, The London School of Economics & Political Science, *Observer* (18 June 2006).

5 Confidential Enquiry into Maternal and Child Health, www.cemach.org.uk

6 Oates, M., 'Perinatal psychiatric disorders: a leading cause of maternal morbidity and mortality', *British Medical Bulletin*, Vol 67 (2003), pp. 219–29.

7 *The Depression Report: A New Deal for Depression and Anxiety Disorders*, A report by The Centre for Economic Performance's Mental Health Policy Group, The London School of Economics & Political Science, *Observer* (18 June 2006).

8 *The Times* (19 November 2007).

9 *The Times* (Supplement) (27 November 2007).

10 David Servan-Schreiber, *Healing without Freud or Prozac*, Rodale International (2005).

11 Anjana Ahuja, 'Sadness, a natural antidote', *The Times* (3 December 2007).

12 'Ditch the pills', *New Scientist* (23 July 2005).

13 van Praag, H.M., 'Why has the antidepressant era not shown a significant drop in suicide rates?' www.biopsychiatry.com/suicide.html

14 Gray, P., 'Biochemical imbalance in the brain – does it exist?' *Therapy Today*, Vol 18(8) (Oct 2007).

15 Rose Shepherd, 'Is your medicine loaded?' *Sunday Times Magazine* (31 July 2005).

16 Tipler, P., *Physics for scientists and engineers: electricity, magnetism, light and elementary modern physics*, 5th edition, W.H. Freemen (2004).

17 Christine Toomey and Steven Young, 'Mental Cruelty', *Sunday Times Magazine* (19 February 2006).

18 Corsellis, J. and Meyer, A., 'Histological changes in the brain after uncomplicated electro-convulsive treatment', *J Mental Sci*, Vol 100 (1954), pp. 375–83; Ebaugh, F.G., et al, 'Fatalities following electric convulsive therapy. A report of two cases with autopsy findings', *Trans Am Neurol Assoc*, Vol 36 (1942); Ferraro, A., et al, 'Morphologic changes in the brains of monkeys following convulsions electrically induced', *J Neuropathol Exp Neurol*, Vol 5 (1946), p. 285; Janis, I.L., 'Psychologic effects of electric convulsive treatments. I: Post-treatment amnesias', *J Nervous Mental Dis*, Vol 111 (1950), pp. 359–81.

19 Amen, D.G., *Neuropsychiatry*, Vol 2(1) (2001), www.neuropsychiatryreviews.com/feb01/npt_feb01_spect.html

20 Dobbs, D., 'Eric Kandel: From mind and brain and back again', *Scientific American Mind*, Vol 33 (November 2007), pp. 33–7.

21 Lechin, F., Vanden Dijs, B. and Lechin, M.E., *Neurocircuitry and Neuroautonomic Disorders*, Karger (2002).

22 Dobbs, D., 'Turning off Depression', *Scientific American Mind* (2006).

23 Cited in www.personeltoday.com

24 Basant Puri, *Attention-Deficit Hyperactivity Disorder: a natural way to treat ADHD*, Hammersmith Press (2005).

25 Park, M., et al, 'Consumption of milk and calcium in midlife and the future risk of Parkinson disease', *Neurology*, Vol 64 (2005), pp. 1047–51; 'Dairy linked to dementia', *Veggiehealth*, issue 14 (summer 2007), p. 8 (quoting work by M.E. Payne).

26 *The Depression Report: A New Deal for Depression and Anxiety Disorders*, A report by The Centre for Economic Performance's Mental Health Policy Group, the London School of Economics & Political Science.

The 12 Golden Guidelines

1 Jane Plant and Gill Tidey, *Eating for Better Health*, Virgin Books (2005).

Resources

For updates and further information regarding support, please visit www.janeplant.com and www.stress-anxiety-depression-support.com

MENTAL HEALTH CHARITIES

Association for Post-Natal Illness
www: apni.org
145 Dawes Road
Fulham
London SW6 7EB
helpline: 020 7386 0868
Provides support for mothers with post-natal depression.

Bipolar Fellowship Scotland
www.bipolarscotland.org.uk
Studio 1016
Mile End Mill
Abbeymill Business Centre
Seedhill Road
Paisley PA1 1TJ
tel: 0141 560 2050

Depression Alliance
www.depressionalliance.org
e-mail: information@depressionalliance.org
212 Spitfire Studios
63–71 Collier Street
London N1 9BE
tel: 0845 123 2320
This charity provides support for those affected by depression and their carers. Its website includes information on its campaigns, local support groups and includes a glossary of illnesses and treatments.

Equilibrium: The Bipolar Foundation
www.bipolar-foundation.org
1 Rivercourt
1 Trinity Street
Oxford OX1 1TQ
This is an independent research organisation looking at the treatment, causes and effects of bipolar disorder at an international level. It has information about the condition and resources for people with bipolar disorder, their family and friends.

ISAD (International Society for Affective Disorders)
www.isad.org.uk
e-mail: enquiry@isad.org.uk; help@isad.org.uk
Institute of Psychiatry
King's College
PO Box 72 De Crespigny Park
Denmark Hill
London SE5 8AF
tel: 020 7848 0295
This is a user-led, registered charity based in East London that is aimed at developing an 'International Perspective of Depression', including unipolar and bipolar depression and generalised anxiety disorder. It aspires to become the principal international, non-profit making society for the advancement and promotion of research into the affective disorders through all relevant scientific disciplines.

Manic Depressive Fellowship: The BiPolar Organisation (MDF)
www.mdf.org.uk
e-mail: mdf@mdf.org.uk
Castle Works
21 St George's Road
London SE1 6ES
Tel: 08456 340 540 (UK only) or 020 7793 2600

MDF The BiPolar Organisation Cymru

www.mdfwales.org.uk
e-mail: info@mdfwales.org.uk
22–29 Mill Street
City of Newport
South Wales NP20 5HA
helpline: 08456 340 080
tel: 01633 244244

The BiPolar Organisation is a user-led charity covering England and Wales which helps people affected by bipolar disorder/manic depression to take control of their lives.

Mind

www.mind.org.uk
e-mail: contact@mind.org.uk
15–19 Broadway
London E15 4BQ
tel: 020 8519 2122
Mind info line: 0845 766 0163

Mind Cymru

3rd Floor
Quebec House
Castlebridge
5–19 Cowbridge Road East
Cardiff CF11 9AB
tel: 029 2039 5123

Mind is one of the UK's leading mental health charities and provides a legal service and information as well as contact information for more than 200 local Mind groups which offer community support for service users. Its website includes details of its campaigns and policy briefings.

National Phobics Society
www.phobics-society.org.uk
e-mail: support@phobics-society.org.uk
information: info@phobics-society.org.uk
Zion Community Resource Centre
339 Stretford Road
Hulme
Manchester M15 4ZY
tel: 08444 775 774
A UK charity for sufferers and ex-sufferers of anxiety disorders, including panic disorder. Includes self-help information packs, therapy tapes and online and phone counselling.

ORHP (Office of Rural Health Policy)
www.ruralhealth.hrsa.gov
Health Resources and Services Administration
5600 Fisher's Lane
9A–55 Rockville
MD20857
USA
tel: +1 301 443 0835
The ORHP funds research activities at eight rural health research centres into depression and generalised anxiety disorder (GAD). Because virtually all rural countries have a shortage of mental health professionals, rural residents are less likely to receive services.

The PHI (Healthcare Trust: changing the world of healthcare, forever)
www.phihealth.org.uk
e-mail: info@phihealth.org.uk
22 Higher Spring Gardens
Ottery St Mary
Devon EX11 1HW
tel: 01404 811 131

Rethink Serious Mental Illness
www.rethink.org
information: info@rethink.org
advice: advice@rethink.org
Rethink Head Office
5th Floor
Royal London House
22–25 Finsbury Square
London EC2A 1DX
tel: 0845 456 0455
helpline: 020 8974 6814
Formerly the National Schizophrenia Fellowship, Rethink is the largest voluntary sector provider of mental health services in the UK. The charity provides support to, and campaigns on behalf of, people with a severe mental illness, their carers and families. Its website contains details on its carer and user support groups as well as consultation papers and policy briefings.

Sainsbury Centre for Mental Health
www.scmh.org.uk
e-mail: contact@scmh.org.uk
134–138 Borough High Street
London SE1 1LB
tel: 020 7827 8300
The Sainsbury Centre is a charity that aims to influence national mental health policy and practice through a co-ordinated programme of research, service development and training. Its main areas of concern are acute hospital care, assertive outreach, crisis resolution and primary care. Its website includes discussion forums, publications and analysis.

Samaritans
www.samaritans.org
e-mail: jo@samaritans.org
Chris
PO Box 9090
Stirling FK8 2SA
tel: 08457 909 090 (UK) or 1850 609 090 (Ireland)

SANE

www.sane.org.uk

e-mail: info@sane.org.uk

SANEmail: sanemail@sane.org.uk

1st Floor

Cityside House

40 Adler Street

London E1 1EE

tel: 020 7375 1002

SANEline: 0845 767 8000

SANE is a leading mental health charity (formerly Schizophrenia, A National Emergency) which campaigns for improved rights for mental health users and their carers. Its website includes SANEline, the national mental health helpline, discussion forums and information on the SANE research centre.

Scottish Association for Mental Health (SAMH)

www.samh.org.uk

e-mail: enquire@samh.org.uk

Cumbrae House

15 Carlton Court

Glasgow G5 9JP

tel: 0141 568 7000

This is the leading mental health charity in Scotland, campaigning for greater understanding of mental distress and better hospital and community services. It runs supported accommodation and employment training.

Triumph Over Phobia

www.topuk.org

PO Box 3760

Bath

tel: 0845 600 9601

National UK network of self-help groups dedicated to helping phobia sufferers, including those with agoraphobia, overcome their fear.

PROFESSIONAL BODIES

British Association for Counselling and Psychotherapy
www.bacp.co.uk
e-mail: bacp@bacp.co.uk
BACP
BACP House
15 St John's Business Park
Lutterworth
Leicestershire
LE17 4HB

The British Psychological Society
www.bps.org.uk
e-mail: enquiry@bps.org.uk
St Andrew's House
48 Princess Road East
Leicester LE1 7DR
tel: 0116 254 9568
The BPS is the representative body for psychologists in the UK and aims to encourage scientific discipline in the profession by raising standards of training and practice. Its website includes details of research, reports and conferences.

Royal College of Psychiatrists (RCP)
www.rcpsych.ac.uk
e-mail: rcpsych@rcpsych.ac.uk
17 Belgrave Square
London SW1X 8PG
tel: 020 7235 2351
The professional body for psychiatrists in the UK produces public information on common mental health problems and treatments and runs the Changing Minds campaign which is aimed at reducing the stigma of mental illness.

LABORATORIES AND CLINICS

Acumen
e-mail: acumenlab@hotmail.co.uk
PO Box 129
Tiverton
Devon EX16 0AJ

Amen Clinics
www.amenclinics.com
4019 Westerly Place
Newport Beach
CA 92660
USA
tel: +1 949 266 3700

Biolab
www.biolab.co.uk
e-mail: info@biolab.co.uk
Biolab Medical Unit
The Stone House
9 Weymouth Street
London W1W 6DB
tel: 020 7636 5959/5905

Neuro-Lab
Neuro-Lab Ltd
681 Wimborne Road
Bournemouth
Dorset BH9 2AT

The Doctors Laboratory (TDL)
www.tdlpathology.com
e-mail: tdlpathology.com
60 Whitfield Street
London W1T 4EU
tel: 020 7307 7373
The largest independent provider of clinical laboratory diagnostic services in the UK.

NUTRITIONAL TREATMENT AND INFORMATION

The British Association for Nutritional Therapy (BANT)
www.bant.org.uk
27 Old Gloucester Street
London WC1N 3XX
tel/fax: 08706 061 284
A professional body for nutritional therapists. Members of the public wishing to find a local nutritional therapist can use its online directory to locate a practitioner.

The Brain Bio Centre
www.brainbiocentre.com
London-based outpatient treatment centre of the Food for the Brain Foundation, putting the optimum nutrition approach into practice for those with mental health problems, including depression, learning difficulties, dyslexia, ADHD, autism, schizophrenia, dementia and Alzheimer's.

The Institute for Optimum Nutrition (ION)
www.ion.ac.uk
Avalon House
72 Lower Mortlake Road
Richmond
Surrey TW9 2JY
tel: 020 8614 7800
Runs courses in nutrition, from one-day workshops to a three-year Nutrition Consultants Diploma course that includes training in the optimum nutrition approach to mental health. They have a clinic, a list of nutrition practitioners across the UK, an information service and a quarterly journal – *Optimum Nutrition*.

Food for the Brain
www.foodforthebrain.org
An educational charity to promote the link between optimum nutrition and mental health. It has a free mental health e-news service, a library of new research and special reports and free online Mental Health Questionnaire and Food for the Brain Child Questionnaire which can help you identify imbalances correctable by optimum nutrition.

Food and Behaviour Research
www.fabresearch.org
Charitable organisation dedicated both to advancing scientific research into the links between nutrition and human behaviour and to making the findings from such research available to the widest possible audience. They have an excellent website and a free e-news service. Sign up at www.fabresearch.org.

The Food and Mood Project
www.foodandmood.org
The aim of this project is to empower individuals to explore the relationship between diet, nutrition and emotional and mental health, and to share this information with others. They have a quarterly newsletter, hold conferences and work closely with Mind to help improve awareness of the links between nutrition and mental health problems.

STRESS REDUCTION: T'AI CHI, YOGA, MEDITATION

The London School of T'ai Chi Chuan and Traditional Health Resources
http://taichi.gn.apc.org/
PO Box 98836
London SE3 0ZG
tel: 020 8566 1677

Taoist T'ai Chi Society of Great Britain
www.taoist-tai-chi-gb.org/
Bounstead Road
Blackheath
Colchester
Essex CO2 0DE
tel: 01206 576167

The British Wheel of Yoga
office@bwy.org.uk
tel: 01529 306851
Supplies information on local classes.

Iyengar Yoga Institite at Maida Vale
www.iyi.org.uk
e-mail: office@iyi.org.uk
223a Randolph Avenue
London W9 1NL
tel: 020 7624 3080
They can put you in touch with Iyengar teachers both in the UK and around the world.

Siddha Yoga Meditation
www.syduk.org
The Amadeus Centre
50 Shirland Road
Little Venice
London W9 2JA
national enquiry line: 01404 514403
Offers one-day courses in meditation and free weekly meditation programmes at its London Centre.

The London Buddhist Centre
www.lbc.org.uk
e-mail: info@lbc.org.uk
51 Roman Road
London E2 0HU
tel: 0845 458 4716
Offers meditation programmes and courses.

OTHER USEFUL ORGANISATIONS

Alcoholics Anonymous
www.alcoholics-anonymous.org.uk
helpline: 0845 769 7555

Association of Reflexologists
www.aor.org.uk
e-mail: info@aor.org.uk
5 Fore Street
Taunton
Somerset TA1 1HX
tel: 01823 351010

The British Acupuncture Council (BAcC)
www.acupuncture.org.uk
e-mail: info@acupuncture.org.uk
63 Jeddo Road
London W12 9HQ
tel: 020 8735 0400

British Register of Complementary Medicine (ICM-BRCP)

www.i-c-m.org.uk

PO Box 194

London SE16 1QZ

tel: 020 7237 5165

Professional register of practitioners who have proved their competence to practise by either completing an approved course or through an assessment made by the Registration Panel. They also agree to abide by a Code of Ethics and Practice and have full practitioner insurance.

ChildLine

www.childline.org.uk

Freepost NATN1111

London E1 6BR

tel: 0800 1111

Childline is a free helpline for children and young people in the UK, who can call 24 hours a day and talk to counsellors about any problem.

Citizens' Advice Bureau

www.citizensadvice.org.uk

The main website will help you to find your nearest office; alternatively consult your telephone directory. For general advice and frequently asked questions try logging on to: www.adviceguide.org.uk.

Cruse Bereavement Care

www.crusebereavementcare.org.uk/

e-mail: info@cruse.org.uk; helpline@cruse.org.uk

PO Box 800

Richmond

Surrey TW9 1RG

helpline: 0844 477 9400

tel: 020 8939 9530

Northern Ireland Regional Office
e-mail: northern.ireland@cruse.org.uk
Piney Ridge
Knockbracken Healthcare Park
Saintfield Road
Belfast BT8 8BH
tel: 028 9079 2419

Cruse Bereavement Care Cymru
e-mail: wales.cymru@cruse.org.uk
Ty Energlyn
Heol Las
Caerphilly/ Caerffili CF83 2TT
tel: 029 2088 6913

Food Standards Agency
www.food.gov.uk

MAMA (Meet-A-Mum Association)
www.mama.co.uk
helpline: 0845 120 3746

Mental Health Act Commission
www.mhac.org.uk
Maid Marion House
56 Hound's Gate
Nottingham NG1 6BG
tel: 0115 943 7100
This watchdog is a special health authority fully independent of mental health service providers. Its main function is to review the operation of the Mental Health Act 1983 in relation to detained patients. Its website offers best practice guidance and legal advice for patients on consent for treatment, including how to have their detention reviewed.

Mental Health Alliance
www.mentalhealthalliance.org.uk
e-mail: gayle.killilea@scmh.org.uk
c/o SCMH
134–138 Borough High Street
London SE1 1LB
tel: 020 7716 6782
This is a coalition of more than 50 service user and provider organisations who share common concerns about the government's draft bill to reform the 1983 Mental Health Act. The website contains press releases, briefing papers, reports and details of events and links to articles on the Alliance's work and aims.

Mental Health Special Interest Group (MHSIG)
www.basw.co.uk
e-mail: info@basw.co.uk
c/o British Association of Social Workers
16 Kent Street
Birmingham B5 6RD
tel: 0121 622 3911
This is a subgroup of the British Association of Social Workers. Its website includes policy briefings, news, reports and response to proposed reforms of the Mental Health Act.

Narcotics Anonymous
www.ukna.org
e-mail: NAHelpline@ukna.org
helpline: 0845 373 3366

National Childbirth Trust
www.nct.org.uk
Alexandra House
Oldham Terrace
Acton
London W3 6NH
tel: 0870 444 8707

National Institute for Health and Clinical Excellence (NICE)
www.nice.org.uk/
e-mail: nice@nice.org.uk
MidCity Place
71 High Holborn
London WC1V 6NA
tel: 020 7067 5800

National Institute of Medical Herbalists
www.nimh.org.uk
e-mail: nimh@ukexeter.freeserve.co.uk
Elm House
54 Mary Arches Street
Exeter EX4 3BA
tel: 01392 426022

Soil Association
www.soilassociation.org
South Plaza
Marlborough Street
Bristol BS1 3NX
tel: 0117 314 5000

Soil Association Scotland
e-mail: contact@sascotland.org
18 Liberton Brae
Tower Mains
Edinburgh EH16 6AE
tel: 0131 666 2474

WEBSITES

For the many useful sites on mental health, contact:
www.guardian.co.uk/society/health

The BBC has produced a PDF booklet on bipolar disorder called 'The Secret Life of Manic Depression: Everything You Need to Know about

Bipolar Disorder'. If you're looking for comprehensive information, download the booklet from:

www.bbc.co.uk/health/tv_and_radio/secretlife_index.shtml

It takes a detailed look at the symptoms and diagnosis of the condition, medical treatments and how to self-manage the condition successfully. First published in 2000, reviewed in 2006.

The Department of Health

www.dh.gov.uk

This website has lots of information on mental health, including a directory of legislation, policy, research, practice, therapies and services. The site also contains information on the Mental Health Act 1983.

Hyperguide to the Mental Health Act

www.hyperguide.co.uk/mha/

An overview of current mental health legislation in England and Wales. It is a good reference source for mental health professionals and service users. The 1983 Mental Health Act governs the admission of people to psychiatric hospital against their will, their rights while detained, discharge from hospital, and aftercare.

The Institute of Psychiatry, the **Maudsley NHS Trust** and the charity **Rethink** together have a website www.mentalhealthcare.org.uk with a comprehensive section on bipolar disorder.

Useful US sites

Agoraphobics Building Independent Lives (ABIL)

www.mhav.org/programs.html

Non-profit organisation providing support and education for those suffering from panic attacks, agoraphobia and phobias. Includes a network of self-help groups, articles on anxiety and book reviews.

Agoraphobia Insight

www.anxietyinsight.com

Guide to agoraphobia and its treatment. Find answers to frequently asked questions, an overview of causes, and a list of common symptoms.

Agoraphobia and Panic Disorder Foundation

www.paniccure.com

Overcoming Agoraphobia – step-by-step guide to overcoming agoraphobia. Describes helpful cognitive techniques, how to create 'safe bases outside the home', and what to do if you have a panic attack while practising.

Anxieties.com

www.anxieties.com

Free self-help site for people with anxiety disorders, including panic disorder. Features a self-assessment questionnaire, weekend treatment groups, and a 'Don't Panic Self-Help Kit'.

Anxiety Disorders Association of America (ADAA)

www.adaa.org

Non-profit organisation dedicated to the diagnosis, treatment and cure of anxiety disorders. Provides a newsletter, a national network of self-help groups in the USA, and a search tool for finding a therapist.

AnxietyPanic.com

www.anxietypanic.com

Site dedicated to educating patients, families, carers and the community about anxiety and panic disorders.

Freedom from Fear

www.freedomfromfear.org

e-mail: help@freedomfromfear.org

National non-profit mental health advocacy association dedicated to helping depression and anxiety sufferers, including those with panic disorder and agoraphobia.

Helpguide.org

www.helpguide.org

Panic attack and agoraphobia discussion forum – register to join and participate in this free online discussion forum focusing on panic disorder and agoraphobia.

The Panic Agoraphobia Support Group
www.geocities.com/Heartland/Estates/1225/support/
Online support group for people with panic disorder and agoraphobia. Features an e-mail list, educational resources and creative writing by members.

AUSTRALIA

Limelight Foundation
www.limelight.org.au
e-mail: info@limelight.org.au
117b Henley Beach Road
Mile End
South Australia 5031
tel: +61 1300 765 997
This not-for-profit organisation offers support services associated with depression, anxiety, mental disorders and stress related issues. Its outlook is to be involved with the community, metropolitan and rural, in battling mental disorders.

Mental Health Council of Australia
www.mhca.org.au
e-mail: admin@mhca.org.au
This national non-governmental organisation represents and promotes the interests of the Australian mental health sector. Members include representatives of mental health service consumers, carers, special needs groups, clinical service providers, public and private mental health service providers and state/territory mental health peak bodies.
Alia House
1st Floor, 9–11 Napier Close
Deakin, ACT 2600
tel: +61 (0)2 6285 3100

SANE Australia
www.sane.org
e-mail: info@sane.org
This charity works for a better life for people affected by mental illness
through campaigns, education and research.
PO Box 226
South Melbourne
Victoria 3205
tel: +61 (0)3 9682 5933

NEW ZEALAND

Mental Health Foundation
www.mentalhealth.org.nz
e-mail: resource@mentalhealth.org.nz
This foundation works to enable individuals, organisations and communities to improve and sustain their mental health and realise their
full potential.
81 New North Road
Eden Terrace
Auckland 1021
tel: +64 (0)9 300 7010

Balance
www.balance.org.nz
e-mail: info@balance.org.nz
PO Box 13266
Armagh
Christchurch 8141
tel: +64 (0)3 366 3631
This organisation provides support, education, advocacy and training
to people affected by bipolar disorder or depression in New Zealand.

Like Minds
www.likeminds.org.nz
tel: +64 (0)800 102 107
This is a public health funded project that aims to reduce the stigma of mental illness and the discrimination that people with experience of mental illness face everyday in the community. There are 26 regional Like Minds providers around the country that undertake a wide variety of anti-discrimination activities within their local communities, businesses and their local media.

SOUTH AFRICA

Mental Health Information Centre
www.mentalhealthsa.co.za
e-mail: mhic@sun.ac.za
Mental Health Information Centre
Room 0068, Clinical Building
University of Stellenbosch Tygerberg Campus
tel: +27 (0)21 938 9229
This charity deals with all kinds of psychiatric disorders, such as Alzheimers, Anxiety Disorder, Bipolar Disorder, Epilepsy, and many more mental illnesses.

South African Depression and Anxiety Group
www.sadag.co.za
e-mail: zane1@hargray.com
tel: +27 (0)11 783 1474
This charity provides free confidential and supportive telephone counselling and has initiated rural development projects in communities where little or no mental health care services are available.

Post-Natal Support Association
www.pndsa.co.za
e-mail: info@pndsa.org.za
tel: +27 (0)82 882 0072
This non-profit organisation provides information and support for women from all walks of life who are experiencing Postnatal Depression, and their families, in order to ensure early identification, timely referral and effective treatment.

PUBLICATIONS

Amen, Daniel G. and Routh, Lisa C., *Healing Anxiety and Depression*, Health 7 & Fitness, Berkeley Publishing Group (2004).
Healing Anxiety and Depression reveals the major anxiety and depression centres of the brain, and offers guidelines and diagnostic tools.

Beck, C. T., 'The effects of postpartum depression on maternal–infant interaction: a meta-analysis', *Nursing Research*, Vol 44 (1995), pp. 298–304 .

Bourne, Edmund, *The Anxiety and Phobic Workbook*, New Harbinger Publications (2000).
Offers help with anxiety, especially for panic attacks.
Gilbert, Paul, *Overcoming Depression: A Step by Step Approach to Gaining Control Over Depression*, Oxford University Press (1997).
'If you suffer from depression, you are, sadly, far from being alone ...'
Gilbert offers depressed people a course of action to change the way they think themselves and their problems.

Greenberger, Dennis and Padesky, Christine, *Mind over Mood: Change the Way You Feel by Changing the Way You Think*, Guilford Press (1995).

Holford, Patrick, *Patrick Holford's New Optimum Nutrition for the Mind*, Piatkus (2007).

James, Oliver, *They Fuck You Up: How To Survive Family Life*, Bloomsbury (2003).
By understanding the effects of the way we were brought up in the first six years of life, James gives us insights as to how to change the way we are.

Luciani, Joseph J., *Self-Coaching: How to Heal Anxiety and Depression*, John Wiley (2006).
Nearly everyone has suffered from mild anxiety or depression at some point in his or her life.

Murray, L. and Cooper, P.J., 'The impact of postpartum depression on child development', *International Review of Psychiatry*, Vol 8 (1996), pp. 55–63.

Puri, Professor Bassant K., *Attention-Deficit Hyperactivity Disorder*, Hammersmith Press (2005).
Helps the reader understand the chemistry of the brain and the many factors that influence it.

Servan-Schreiber, Dr David, *Healing Without Freud or Prozac*, Rodale International (2005).
Natural approaches to curing stress, anxiety and depression. It shows you how to tap into the emotional brain's self-healing process.

Wheatley, Sandra, *Coping with Postnatal Depression*, Sheldon Press (2005).

Wolpert, Lewis, *Malignant Sadness, The Anatomy of Depression*, Faber & Faber (2006).
Wolpert, a professor of biology as applied to medicine, shares his own experience of depression.

Yield, Jenny (ed.), *Cognition, Emotion and Psychopathology: Theoretical, Experimental and Clinical Directories*, University of Oxford (2004).
It presents a 'state of the art' account of the cognitive-clinical literature and sets an agenda for future work.

Index

Note: page numbers in **bold** refer to diagrams.

About the Authors

PROFESSOR JANE PLANT is the author of the international bestseller *Your Life in Your Hands*, which explains how she overcame advanced breast cancer by complementing her medical treatment with dietary and lifestyle changes. Professor Plant is a Professor of Environmental Geochemistry at Imperial College, London, and has been awarded a CBE for services to earth sciences.

JANET STEPHENSON is a psychologist who works as a therapist within the NHS and in private practice. For the last ten years she has been part of a hospital specialist team tackling drug and alcohol addiction.